Tao Shiatsu

Tao Shiatsu

Life Medicine for the Twenty-First Century

Ryokyu Endo

Foreword by Robert Bosnack

Japan Publications, Inc.

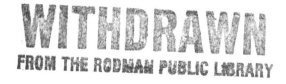

© 19

Forev

Trans

Photographs by Task Hamazaki

Illustrations by Masaru Domoto and Keiko Koiwa

Design, typesetting and layout by Jerald Volpe, the BOOKWORKS

Note to the reader: Those with health problems are advised to seek the guidance of a qualified medical or psychological professional before implementing any of the approaches presented in this book. It is essential that any readers who have any reason to suspect serious illness in themselves or their family members seek appropriate medical, nutritional, or psychological advice promptly. Neither this nor any other health-related books should be used as a substitute for qualified care or treatment.

Published by

JAPAN PUBLICATIONS, INC., Tokyo and New York

JAPAN PUBLICATIONS TRADING CO., LTD., Tokyo and Brisbane

Distributors:

United States: Kodansha America, Inc., through Farrar, Straus & Giroux, 19 Union Square West, New York, N.Y. 10003. *Canada:* Fitzhenry & Whiteside Ltd., 195 Allstate Parkway, Markham, Ontario L3R 4T8. *British Isles and European Continent:* Premier Book Marketing Ltd., 1 Gower Street, London WC1E 6HA. *Australia and New Zealand:* Bookwise International, 54 Crittenden Road, Findon, South Australia 5023. *The Far East and Japan:* Japan Publications Trading Co., Ltd., 1-2-1, Sarugaku-cho, Chiyoda-ku, Tokyo 101.

First Edition: January 1995

ISBN 0-87040-940-9

Printed in the United States of America

Contents

Foreword   vii

Introduction — Why Study Tao Shiatsu Now?   1

    Medicine, Culture, and Environment   2
    Yin and Yang   9
    The Eastern View of Life   18
    The Role of Tao Shiatsu in the Twenty-First Century   26

Chapter 1 — *Ki* and Shiatsu Healing Techniques   31

    What is *Ki?*   32
    Ki and Image   40
    Doin-Ankyo and the Art of Immortality   49
    Teate: Touch Therapy   54

Chapter 2 — Basic Techniques   61

    The Various Techniques of Shiatsu   62
    The Three Principles of Shiatsu   70
    The Principles of the *Ki* Shiatsu Method   84
    The Basic Forms of Tao Shiatsu   90
    Shiatsu for Children   121

Chapter 3 — *Sho* Diagnosis   141

    What Is *Sho*?   142
    Perceiving *Sho*   154
    Techniques of Meridianal Diagnosis   157

Chapter 4 — Meridians   167

    Meridians and the Body   168
    Six, Twelve, and Twenty-Four Meridians   173
    The *Kyo-Jitsu* Pattern in the Meridians   178
    The Twenty-Four Meridians throughout the Body   191

Chapter 5 — Meridianal Therapy   221

    Tsubo and Meridians   222
    The Practice of Meridianal Therapy   229

The Philosophy of Meridianal Therapy   237
The Menken Response   242
Diagnosis in Chinese Medicine   246

Epilogue   255

Glossary   259

Index   261

Foreword

When we first came to Japan in 1985 at the invitation of Hayao Kawai, my wife was recuperating from a serious car accident she had suffered several months previously. She had been in the hospital for a week with pains that could not be diagnosed. Finally, after a series of expensive, extensive, and invasive tests, an x-ray revealed that a kidney had been bruised and nothing further could be done. It would just take time to heal. When we arrived in Tokyo after our long trip from Boston, my wife again suffered pain, and we asked our host, who had invited me to teach dream seminars in Japan, to find us a therapist in Oriental medicine. Into our room at the International House in Tokyo came a highly recommended young man, Ryokyu Endo, who checked her abdomen and concluded in thirty seconds that my wife had damaged a kidney. After one hour of shiatsu treatment, the pains never returned (knock on wood).

On one of my yearly teaching visits since, I was plagued by a serious backache, an ailment that had afflicted me regularly since the age of twenty-three. When I arrived in Kyoto I could hardly walk. Endo touched a point in my right thigh after some other manipulations, put on a certain amount of pressure, looking inward and detached while doing so, and I have not worn a back brace for over a year since. But Ryokyu Endo's work is not magic. He is just very good at what he does and knows the body from within, how to follow the subtle flow of life pulsating through us by way of rivers of vitality called meridians.

His book is eminently practical, which would be praise enough. It shows how *ki*, the life force felt by the East in all its many differentiations since prehistoric times, is manifested and can be influenced. The Orient places the highest value on felt experience as a primary source of knowledge. Rational expression and description are secondary. Reproduction of the experience is the motive for writing, more than the dissemination of academic knowledge. In this way Ryokyu Endo is a capable communicator. Having lived in the West as a youth for several years, he knows his audience beyond his homeland. He is easy to understand for Westerners. If you want to learn a new way of treatment, this is your book. Not only is the philosophy sound, but the many illustrations and specific manipulations are graphic and clear. If you want to experience a world that never labored under the illusion of a distinct separation of body and soul, learn from this young master who knows how to heal. During the last few years Ryokyu Endo has concentrated his efforts on disseminating his method by training many therapists. The fact that he is now primarily an instructor greatly enhances the clarity of this book. Endo is a gifted musician as well, composing meditative music, recorded on compact disc. His meditative musical mind plays through all pages of the book.

As a psychoanalyst specializing in the work on dreams, I am well aware of the intimate relationship between psyche and body. This relationship comes through images that engender physical responses. Endo's use of these images is masterful, and I trust this book will increase the understanding in the West of an Oriental state of mind that trusts human intuition as a primary tool in the acquisition of knowledge.

— Robert Bosnak,
author of *A Little Course in Dreams*
and *Dreaming with an AIDS Patient*

Introduction

Why Study
Tao Shiatsu Now?

Medicine, Culture, and Environment

Nature: Obedience in the East and Manipulation in the West

Oriental medicine, whether it is shiatsu, acupuncture, or Chinese herbal medicine, cures illness by guiding the patient's natural energies. According to the philosophy of Oriental medicine, illness appears when the body loses its harmony with nature because the alternating currents of energy between the patient and nature are obstructed. Treatment consists of stimulating the dormant vital energy in the patient and restoring its circulation to normal. Appropriate treatment varies according to the individual patient's vital response. In order to stimulate this healing response, the therapist must work in harmony with the patient's life energies. The therapist is then able to act as mediator in restoring the patient's harmony with nature, which will eventually take over the healing process altogether. Because the goal of therapeutic techniques in Oriental medicine is this self-healing response, treatment is basically performed by human hands rather than machines or implements. Furthermore, therapies that rely on this sympathetic response can only be determined by a diagnosis that is also carried out by human hands.

In the East, nature's powers have traditionally been considered precious and sacred. Some of the distinctive features of Oriental medicine are the absence of drugs and machinery and the absence of focus on any one part of the body. Medical treatment is approached through gentle, natural methods. Shiatsu is said to be the most natural manual technique and plays a central role in the different therapies of Oriental medicine. The Eastern concept of nature as master is understood when dealing with disease and treatment in Oriental medicine, which perceives the essence of life from the point of view of a mutual exchange with nature. Treatment that emphasizes harmony with nature and faithful obedience toward nature is based on the philosophy that nurtured the cultures of the East. As such it is inconceivable to separate Oriental medicine from the natural features of the Eastern lands.

Owing to its warm climate, high rainfall, and fertile soils, the East has long been a well-established agricultural society. Blessed with such a mild climate, Eastern peoples have not needed an ideology placing the self in opposition with nature. In contrast, the European environment is harsh, and, throughout history, its people have had to subjugate natural elements in order to survive.

Europe is located on a higher latitude than most of Japan. Environments in this northern latitude must endure long, cold, harsh winters; understandably, European houses are built from stone to isolate people from their external environment. In contrast, Japanese houses are made of wood with verandas, open corridors, and ambiguous boundaries between the exterior and interior because in Japan, people have not had to isolate themselves from nature in order to survive. If European houses were built with consideration for the winter cold, Japanese houses were built with the same consideration for the hot, humid summers. Japanese summers may be uncomfortable because of high temperatures and humidity, but a positive and important aspect of these climatic conditions is that the country is never without an abundant supply of water.

The European land mass was formed by erosion during the last glacial period and the soil is relatively infertile, making it unsuitable for agriculture. Furthermore, throughout most of Europe, the sunlight is weak; and because there is little precipitation, water is scarce. It is said that if Japanese rice were grown in Europe, the harvested crop would not exceed one fifth of the same crop in Japan. A tree that takes fifty years to grow in Japan takes one hundred fifty years to grow in Germany.[1] On the other hand, the relatively low rainfall in Europe means that weeds are not prolific and the abundant pastures are very suitable for cattle raising, which became the main means of subsistence throughout European history. Continued grazing depletes pastures, however, and the lifestyle of early European communities was structured on a cyclical migratory pattern over a period of several years. Among people who lead such lifestyles there is necessarily a mutually competitive principle at work, and the ensuing definition of boundaries between oneself and others generates disorder and disputes.

---

1. Mitsuo Ishikawa, *Nyu Saiensu no Sekaikan* [in Japanese] (Tokyo: Tama, 1985).

In some parts of Europe, the severity of the climate gave rise to a culture that manipulates nature. Searching for and migrating to land suitable for cattle farming and raising other animals brought about an ideology that placed people as the rulers of nature. Therefore, individuality became an inherent feature of Western psychology. In fact, these aspects of human character are well represented and respected in the New Testament. Therefore, it can be said that the tendency in Western culture to distinguish the subject (the ego) from the object (the physical world) may not be unrelated to the fact that European society is founded on a society based on cattle farming.

Austere spiritual ideologies and religions with rigid commandments are born in lands where a harsh natural environment fosters inflexible beliefs. Lands where the natural features of the environment are lifeless and harsh, such as the desert lands of the world, foster religious beliefs in only one god; for example, Mohammedanism, Christianity, and Judaism. On the other hand, belief in many gods emerges in lands that abound in nature and are rich in seasonal changes, such as the East, where there is natural reverence for the sun, mountains, rivers, and in fact everything in nature. Hinduism in India, Taoism in China, and Shinto in Japan are all polytheistic. Buddhism was born from the belief that even felons can be saved by Amida Buddha and the preaching of the Lotus Sutra, namely that the Buddha Nature exists in everyone and everything.

Western Medicine

Therapeutic techniques in Western medicine are carried out by means of surgical operations or medical drugs, resulting in the invasive manipulation of the patient's body. These techniques are in some ways an obvious consequence of the desire to control nature that is inherent to Western culture. Western medicine treats the body and mind as separate entities. One reason for this is that research on the physical structure of the body began with autopsy. However, more significantly, it is because Western medicine was originally based on natural science, a discipline that studies everything from a purely objective point of view, doing all it can to exclude the subjective mind from research. Furthermore, natural science reduces all things in existence to elements of structure and maintains that the more something is subdivided, the more its true form may be understood, leading Western medicine to view the whole body as a machine made up of different parts.

Another characteristic of Western medicine is the manipulation of the body's natural functions. In cases of chronic illness in particular, all too often the internal functions of the body are diagnosed as being either excessive or deficient. For instance, the cause of diabetes is said to be a deficiency of insulin, Parkinson's disease a deficiency of dopamine. Treatment of such illnesses takes the form of isolating the deficient internal element, chemically synthesizing it externally, and then administering it to the patient. In other words, the deficient element is directly and artificially supplemented. Western medicine has excelled in the area of emergency therapy, and drugs have an immediate effect because they work directly on the physical body. However, when deficiencies are physically supplemented by drugs, the body becomes lazy and loses the ability to produce the deficient element naturally, thereby making it impossible to return to a true condition of health. This situation is profitable for pharmaceutical companies but hardly beneficial for the patient. Long-term dependency on drugs invariably has secondary effects, and even if a medicine is effective for a specific organ, it may damage other organs, which may result in further dependency.

Holistic Medicine

As previously mentioned, people involved in agriculture consider all things in relation to nature as a whole. People in agricultural communities eat from their crops and return their excrement to the land, forming a cycle between themselves and nature. In Oriental medicine, the human body is regarded in the same way as the earth. Every cycle in nature is a function of the circulation of natural energy. Oriental medicine views the human body as one cycle in nature; a miniature universe. Born from this concept, the Theory of the Five Elements of Yin and Yang (chapter 4) explains that the energy cycle of Nature also exists in the human body.

The natural environment greatly influences its inhabitants' view of nature. Even in the West, the Greek philosophical views of the body and nature, born in the temperate climate of the Mediterranean regions, closely resemble those of the East. Chinese philosophy and martial arts are also believed to have originated with reflection on the culture born from the various natural climatic changes inherent in the East. Among the practices of Oriental medicine, established in China thousands of years ago, the ancient Chinese emphasized the manual techniques known as *doin* and *ankyo* (chapter 1). *Doin,* like yoga and *qigong,* is a method of maintaining health through one's own efforts with exercise and breathing techniques. *Ankyo* is a corrective technique that uses manual pressure and the patient's energy. Both techniques came about through what is known as the Rules of Health, which set out to awaken the body and mind to the cosmos.

Doin and *ankyo* occupy a central place in Oriental medicine, emphasizing the assimilation of life with the source of universal consciousness rather than the curing of disease. The medical classics state that curing a disease once it has started is like digging a well when one is thirsty. The Rules of Health are born from the ideal of assimilating oneself with universal consciousness and maintaining the youth of one's mind and body. Unlike Western medicine, which views illness pathologically as a disorder in one part of the body, Oriental medicine perceives illness as an indication of disharmony between nature and humankind. This disharmony is said to be caused by people focusing too much on themselves and becoming unable to respond and adapt to changes in nature. Oriental medicine excludes the patient's ego from treatment and heals by drawing out one hundred percent of the patient's natural inner strength.

This type of medical care is by no means unique to Oriental medicine. Beyond the limits of allopathy is homeopathy, which originated in Germany and cures illness through the patient's physical life responses. Allopathy prescribes medication to lower blood pressure in patients who suffer from high blood pressure. Homeopathy lowers blood pressure by prescribing a minute dose of medication that initially heightens the blood pressure even more. The patient's body then reacts by naturally lowering its own blood pressure. Unlike in modern medicine, where it is necessary to continue taking medication even after the blood pressure is lowered, the positive aspect of homeopathy is that the patient can discontinue medication.

Research on the different pharmacological effects of Chinese medicine reveals some ambiguity, and the pharmacological effects of homeopathic medicine cannot be studied by the analytical techniques of natural science. In particular, the rules of dilution in homeopathic medicine (the more a homeopathic remedy is diluted with water, the greater the therapeutic effect) cannot be expressed in terms of quantity and dosage. Chinese medicine and homeopathic remedies, unlike modern scientific drugs, do not simply have a direct effect on the patient's body. Because these function through a holistic response to the administered dose in the patient's life and body, their effect cannot be measured quantitatively. In Oriental medicine, treatment is basically carried out through this response of the patient's vitality, which is always the object of therapy. The healer does not manipulate the patient's vitality; rather, he or she empathizes with it and always faces his or her patient with an open mind.

In physical and psychiatric medicine, what has recently come to be known as the "therapy of the patient as the subject" has long been considered an ideal in Oriental medicine. This is particularly so in shiatsu therapy. The stimulation of each pressure point in shiatsu therapy is the most fundamental way of empathizing with the patient's vitality. During consultation, the therapist must listen closely and sympathetically to all the patient's complaints and subjective symptoms, because the subject of treatment must always be the patient.

Unlike Western medicine, Oriental medicine does not depend solely on physical attributes. According to the Oriental concept of therapy, the body is furnished with its own natural healing powers; a universal energy that circulates within the patient's living body heals the illness by guiding the patient's natural inner strength. In Oriental medicine, the cause of illness is not simply diagnosed as a deficiency of any particular internal element but as a disorder in the whole body that has stopped production of that element. Therefore, there is no concept or practice of directly supplementing a deficient element in the body. Oriental medicine considers one's immediate environment as a primary cause of disorders in the body. Once the disorder in the patient's whole body has been corrected, the body resumes normal production of any deficient element. Even Chinese herbal medicine has no direct physical effect on the body. It works on the patient's entire energy by stimulating the natural vital strengths that, once redirected, induce a healing response. For example, one known effect of the burn scars from moxibustion on infections is increased production of white blood cells, enabling the body to fight the infection.

Oriental medicine maintains that all life functions through a constant exchange of energy with nature. The body is perceived as a unit, something more than the sum of all its different parts. All parts of the body are understood to have an organic relationship, and each influences the whole body, which functions within an even greater whole: nature. Unlike natural science, Oriental medicine does not acknowledge division between the subject and the object. This is because it is thought that the body can only be understood within the union of both subject and object. This union may be difficult for the novice to understand, but throughout the ages, all doctors who have understood the diagnostic techniques of Oriental medicine have administered therapy and cured illness within the limits of this union. Furthermore, the diagnostic techniques of Oriental medicine cannot be understood outside the psychological boundaries of the union of the subject and object. Based on this unitary concept of the mind and body, Oriental medicine treats the individual and the whole together. This concept of life is acquired by understanding the holistic nature of life and not by dividing it into smaller units and analyzing it, as is the case in Western medicine. Tao shiatsu, which can be considered at the center of Oriental medicine, is based on this concept of life and is said to have originated as a treatment that heals invisible life.

In the temperate climate of the East, nature is respected and obeyed. The culture nurtured there consists of the type of philosophy and art that seeks to harmonize and integrate with nature. Based on a culture generated from such wealth in the natural environment, medical treatment too has arisen from the concept of harmonizing with and obeying nature. Western medicine, on the other hand, has had no perception of harmonizing with nature. Rather, nature has been manipulated to the extent that deteriorating parts of the body may, all too often, be treated by surgical excision.

The philosophy that preaches "non-action in nature" (chapter 1), that is, becoming selfless and entrusting everything to nature, was born in the East with the Oriental agricultural lifestyle as its background. Because a lifestyle that is dependent on agriculture is also dependent on group work, traditionally in the East the tendency has been toward the virtues of the abolition of the ego rather than the development of the individual. Perhaps this is one reason why, compared to Westerners, people in the East do not have a distinct consciousness of the self. Healing by drawing on the natural powers that exist within the patient, and not by artificial manipulation of the patient's body, is one of the characteristics of Oriental medicine, where healers, too, must discard their ego and essentially become one with nature.

The work of people in agricultural communities is to cultivate the soil, sow the seeds, and harvest the crops. But it is the sun, the rain, and the natural powers of the earth that actually ripen the crops. Therefore, the work of the people is to prepare the earth so that it may exhibit its natural inner strength to the maximum. Sowing, harvesting, and all other work done on the land respond to a natural passage of time. Not only medicine but all other aspects of

Eastern culture are based on this compliance with nature. This is not a familiar concept to desert dwellers or people from other harsh environments, because in such climatic and environmental conditions, people must constantly battle with the elements and cannot entrust their livelihood to nature.

Where changes in the seasons are poorly defined, people cannot follow a lifestyle that obeys the cyclic rhythm of nature. Not only is Japan a country where nature is hospitable; it also has four well-defined seasons. Because the environment is blessed with climatic and temporal diversity, the culture that has developed there has been particularly close to, and in harmony with, nature. Changes in the seasons generate the various colors of nature, and variations in the spatial environment enrich people's sensitivity towards nature. Haiku,[2] flower arrangement, the tea ceremony, and all the traditional arts are based on such human sensitivity and are born from a culture that delights in all aspects of nature. In cattle-raising societies, people control other animals, and because meat makes up a large proportion of their diet, people tend to believe they have a special existence that includes the privilege to dominate other animals. However, in agricultural societies where more vegetables are consumed, there is a worldview that all living things are equal; the Buddhist pledge to help all living things is based on this view.

Yin and Yang

The Reciprocal Nature of Yin and Yang

The concept of yin and yang forms the fundamental ideology of Eastern philosophy. Yin and yang are the two mutually contradictory properties of all phenomena. Because yin and yang are explained as the two-sided nature of what is essentially one phenomenon, it is also said that these two polarities

---

2. *Haiku* is seventeen-syllable poetry composed of three lines of five, seven, and five syllables. *Haiku* are traditionally about nature, and each poem contains a subtle expression of the season in which it is written.

are never actually "fixed." Eastern thought does not view differentiation in the natural world (male versus female and so on) antagonistically. Rather, it preaches that all things in creation have a two-sided nature and that Tao, the absolute union of these two sides, exists at the source of the differentiation.

Lao-Tzu preached the following about Tao:

> Tao is something that existed solemnly before the heavens opened. It has no voice and no shape, it is eternal and indestructible, it does not exist in anything, and it is independent of everything. Therefore it may be called the mother of the world, but I don't know what its name could be. So I presumptuously give it the name Tao. When people are not covetous and their minds are clear, they can see the reality of this nameless Tao, but when people are selfish, they always see antagonism and discrimination in the world. The real Tao and the opposition and differentiation in the world are one at their source and everything comes forth from that source as though it were a gate.[3]

Lao-Tzu also preached that Tao is at the source of all things and that in their essence all opposition and differentiations in the world are one with Tao. The I Ching or Book of Changes explains that what existed before the beginning of the universe was *taikyoku*,[4] and that yin and yang were generated and the world began when *taikyoku* moved. Therefore, it is said that yin and yang are generated from one source. Yang is active on the surface of existence while yin exists more deeply as the absolute support of the action of yang. The theory of yin and yang, unlike scientific theory, does not perceive nature as matter. It is an ideology that was born from the intuitive holistic understanding of the existence of "invisible life."

The motivating power behind the development of all creation, and that which contains the opposing properties of yin and yang, is known as *ki* (chapter 1). *Ki* is said to exist as one at its source but has both a dynamic and a restrictive aspect; yang is the dynamic aspect and yin the restrictive. Yin

---

3. Lao-Tzu, pronounced *Roshi* in Japanese, is the founder of Taoist thought. He is believed by some to be a contemporary of Confucius. This is a quote from the Tao Te Ching.
4. *Taikyoku*, pronounced *tai-chi* in Chinese, is primordial polarity. In Chinese philosophy, this is the great void or emptiness from which all life originates. Similar to the Western concept of the Big Bang.

and yang are said to be in a state of change in all natural phenomena because all things in the natural world are born from the existence of opposition and differentiation. The wind blows according to variation in temperature and water flows over the earth according to altitude. New life is born according to sexual differences and cells regenerate according to the dynamics of water pressure in osmosis. This is what is meant by all changes generating from the existence of differentiation. As people, we are able to perceive our own existence because we exist apart from others. We are able to feel heat and cold because there are variations in temperature. In fact all life is conducted by virtue of the existence of such oppositions and differentiations, and all things in the natural world have a reciprocal relationship: woman and man, the positive and negative magnetic poles. Moreover, these polarities cannot exist without their opposite. Similarly, cause and effect are inseparable because each has the potential to be the other. This is known as "simultaneous cause and effect."

Yin and yang are also said to have a "simultaneous cause and effect," and nature is generated by their constant change. The word *I*[5] (from *I Ching*) signifies constant change. Nature is said to exist through change and it is also said to *be* change. Eastern philosophy understands the essence of nature as energy, and because energy is made up of the opposing properties of yin and yang, nature is able to continue to manifest unlimited change. It is with this philosophical background that Oriental medicine understands the body as invisible life or energy and not merely as matter. Therefore, diagnosis in Oriental medicine is not carried out by searching for abnormalities in the physical body and categorizing the illness, but by *sho* diagnosis, which acknowledges the balance and harmony of life and energy (chapter 4).

An example of the manifestation of yin and yang in everyday life can be demonstrated by writing on a blackboard with white chalk. The writing can be seen only because white chalk stands out on the black background. The relationship of the writing and the blackboard is similar to that of yin and yang. Yang is obvious on the surface and can be acknowledged through reasoning. Yin generates yang and maintains the background as a whole. The explanation of yin and yang is by no means limited to the relationship of the chalk and the blackboard. For the contrast is perceived through the sense of sight, and whenever the background is focused on as a whole, the contrast is blurred, whereas when attention is focused on any part, the contrast be-

---

5.   *I*, also pronounced *eki*. Divination, fortune-telling.

comes distinctly clear. Note, for instance, the vase shape created by the black lines in Figure I.1. The black part can be the foundation, in other words the background, allowing the two people facing each other to form the picture, or it may be the picture—the vase—with the white part as the background.

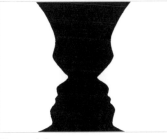

Figure I.1

The manifestations of yin and yang in physical functions may be illustrated by the action of holding a cup in one's hands. We perceive this as one movement, which at first sight seems limited to the muscular function (yang) of the conical system of the upper limbs. In fact, this movement is carried out by the support work of the group of muscles outside the conical system (yin). Yang is obvious as activity on the surface and the existence of yin throughout the body is essential for the background support of its functions. Our conscious actions (yang) are directed by the subconscious (yin). This means that we cannot consciously decide what and how to feel. Furthermore, the conscious and subconscious are different levels of the mind, uniting to form the spiritual energy of the individual. To take the example of the traditional roles of men and women: man, who is yang, is said to be the one involved in making history and providing the functions of society. What is not generally considered is the strength of woman working in the background. Even from a psychological point of view, the social functions of man are strongly supported domestically by the intuitive nature of woman. The true woman can often control man through her own yin energy.

Therefore, although yang is obvious on the surface, it is always entirely sustained by yin in the background. While yin and yang possess these opposing natures and exist in completely different dimensions, each unites with the other to carry out the vital functions of life. The mind is yin and the body is yang, but the life of the individual functions by the union of the two. The body, which has form and weight, and the mind, which is formless and weightless, seem to exist separately, but they are mutually permeable and one at their source. (Therefore, yin and yang have an inseparable relation-ship like the two sides of one coin.) We observe light in exactly the same way: either as particles of matter or as waves. In our natural world all things con-tain the reciprocal nature of yin and yang and are manifested as one phe-nomenon through mutually complementary functions.

Yin and Yang as Light and Shadow: Consciousness and Unconsciousness

Linguistically, yin and yang can be explained as the two sides of a mountain (Figure I.2): one side is that on which the sun shines (yang) while the other side is in shadow (yin). The words *yin* and *yang,* which derive from *shadow* and *sun* respectively, are of the utmost significance in Eastern philosophy, where things that are understood consciously are known as yang and things belonging in the realm of the unconscious are known as yin. People's con-scious actions are likened to the light of the sun because, just as light is nec-essary in order to see, so is consciousness necessary in order to perceive contrast. Behind the things known consciously are those that exist in the realm of the unknown unconscious. What places yin in the realm of the un-conscious is the fact that, inevitably, a shadow is formed on one side of an ob-ject when it is hit by light on the opposite side. In much the same way, in Gestalt psychology, through the contrast created by the picture (yang), the background (yin) on which the picture appears fades away.

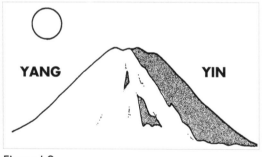

Figure I.2

Is a shadow created by light hitting an object or does the shadow already exist and only become visible because of the light? One may think this is a strange question; but before the sun rises, everything is in darkness. This darkness is, in fact, a shadow. If there were a world where nothing disturbed the existence of light, light could not be recognized as light. We think that shadows exist because light exists, but darkness (or shadow) is essential if we are to recognize light, and light is essential if we are to recognize shadow.

Human consciousness, too, was born through the development of one part of the instinctive mind. Unconsciousness is the root of consciousness, and therefore it cannot be said that consciousness was the first to exist. A newborn infant does not have distinct conscious functions. Children only gradually grow to distinguish between themselves and others, first through the recognition of their mother's existence. Through the development of consciousness of the self, the unconscious is submerged by the conscious, hides behind the conscious, and takes on an earthly existence. In a world completely filled with uniform darkness, the sun rose and created the contrasting phenomena known as light and darkness. Similarly, the child who lives in a world of complete unconsciousness is awakened, through the birth of the light called the "self" or the "ego," to the contrast of the conscious and the unconscious.

With the development of the conscious self, people lapse into the illusion that their consciousness is their master. This is the true form of the self in modern times. Things that cannot be dealt with consciously are buried in the realm of the unconscious, in which case the unconscious exists as the shadow of the conscious. The Western psychologist Carl Jung calls this aspect of the unconscious *the shadow,* and explains that this is the aspect of a person's character that has not been allowed to surface and manifest consciously. For example, the introverted nature of a person who is more extroverted and the extroverted nature of someone who is more introverted are shadow elements. This is why extroverted people often criticize introverted people as lacking the ability to socialize, while introverted people underrate those who are extroverted, feeling they are overly frivolous. Thus, people are disturbed by the hidden sides of their own nature that have not been allowed to surface. Jung called this *projection* (projecting one's own shadow onto someone else).

Jung explains that the self lives through the conceptualization and integration of the unconscious (the shadow) with one's own reality. With clinical evidence and empirical data, he explains that people suffer from nervous disorders when they live only in the conscious world without exceeding the limitations of their own mind. In other words, nervous disorders are said to be caused by the suppressed unconscious asserting its own existence. Therefore, it is very important for people to develop and be in touch with their own subconscious world. Acknowledging the existence of one's whole nature means giving life both to the "normal" conscious world that exists in time and space and to the "abnormal" unconscious world that exists in neither time nor space. Unlike Freud, Jung not only identified the level of emotions suppressed by the superego (known as id) but also the existence of the level of a collective unconscious in the entire human race.

Buddhists believe that the unconscious is divided into several levels, and at the source of the unconscious is the omnipresent, ubiquitous consciousness of the universe, known as the ninth consciousness. In simple terms, the levels of consciousness begin with the six parts of the body that perceive the five senses (eyes, ears, nose, tongue, body, and mind); beyond these is the *mana consciousness.* The English word *man* derives from the Sanskrit word *mana*; it is the "ego" or "self-consciousness," the recognition of the existence of the self. Beyond this is the *alaya vignana* or *alaya consciousness.* The *laya* of *alaya* consciousness means "a place of storage," a place where the power or effect of experiences collects. Another name for *alaya* is what has come to be known as the "collective consciousness."[6] All physical and mental activities are stored together in the *alaya* or collective consciousness, which means that future physical and mental activity is determined by karma, and all incidents that develop in a human lifetime are determined by the *alaya* consciousness. The aim of Buddhist discipline is the purification of the *alaya* consciousness and the awakening of the ninth consciousness, which is the absolute consciousness filled with the love and virtue pervasive in the universe.

Just as the sun rises and casts its light on the mountain, creating a shadow, so too, when people are aware of their own self-consciousness, does the unconscious fall into an existence shadowed by the ego. However, just as everything is in darkness before the sun rises, so too was the world of the vast infinite unconscious, which includes the ninth consciousness, already in people's minds before the awakening to self-consciousness. The ninth consciousness, a universal consciousness that is the source of the unconscious, is directly connected to ubiquitous omnipresent life, and all living things are

---

6. The *hima* of Himalaya means "snow," and because *laya* means a place of storage or collection, the word Himalaya means "a place where snow collects."

born from this source. In the East, more significant consideration is given to intuition, spirituality, and the unconscious, which belong in the realm of yin, than materialism, words, and the conscious, which belong in the realm of yang, because the former has a profound interrelationship with omnipresent life. In Oriental philosophy another name for yin is *emptiness*, from which everything is born and to which everything returns.

Yin and Yang in Medicine and Culture

Yin is the underlying energy of existence, much more closely related to imperceptible phenomena of life than to visible manifestations. Yang pertains to that which can be perceived physically and consciously. Yin belongs in the realm of the whole and yang in individual parts. Oriental medicine, which treats the body and mind as a whole, can be seen as yin medicine, while Western medicine, which treats the body as matter, can be seen as yang medicine. In other words, Oriental medicine acknowledges the holistic nature of the body and mind and treats both as one energy, while Western medicine acknowledges the body and mind as a duality and treats illness as an abnormality of the affected region.

It is not unreasonable to say that the advantages and disadvantages of both Oriental and Western medicine are intensified by treatment of the body as a whole by one, and as individual parts by the other. The differences are similar to one's view of a whole mountain and another's detailed analysis of each tree living on the side of the mountain; a total view of the mountain does not reveal each tree. Because diagnosis in Oriental medicine relies on the healer's intuition, excluding the use of examination equipment and tools, it grasps the holistic condition of the patient's energy but cannot obtain accurate data referring to specific parts of the body. Western medicine considers each tree without seeing the mountain. In other words, even if it is able to grasp the condition of each part of the body, it does not acknowledge the holistic nature of the patient's body and mind, and as such it is inconceivable that it should understand a condition of harmony between the patient and nature.

At present, the main methods of medical treatment throughout the world fall into the categories of either Oriental medicine or Western medicine. Among these, however, the mechanical manipulation of the body, carried out by Western medicine, is generally more accepted than the principles of

Oriental medicine. One cannot say which of the two is ultimately correct. However, it is possible to say that those who think that only one point of view is correct are perhaps focusing on that aspect to an extreme. Because Oriental and Western medicine are yin and yang respectively, each may be understood to be complementary to the other. There are some who believe that since medicine is generally a technique of curing illness, it should be an integration of both Eastern and Western methods. However, as we know, Western medicine does not base its surgical operations on acupuncture and does not prescribe Chinese herbs. Oriental medicine does not place significance on objective acknowledgment of a state of illness and, because its aim is the practice of a different method of therapy for each patient, its scholarly perspective is different from that of Western medicine.

From the point of view of Gestalt psychology, Oriental medicine is the background of the picture in the example mentioned earlier and Western medicine the picture. Western medicine appears to place itself in the foreground by placing Oriental medicine in the background. This does not suggest that Western medicine should incorporate Oriental medicine but that, through making it its foundation, they could both be unified for the first time.

Let us now consider Western culture from the point of view of the theory of yin and yang. All active "things" that have a form that is born and develops are yang, and what fundamentally maintains this activity is yin. When forms of life throughout the planet are viewed from this perspective, animals, which have freedom of movement, are active yang, and plants, which are immobile and have a fundamentally close relationship with the earth, are yin. Yin plants supply yang animals with their source of activity through oxygen and food. In other words, yin maintains yang activity. From this perspective, cultures born from agricultural societies where plants are the staple food are yin, whereas cultures born from cattle-raising societies where animals are the staple food are yang. The agricultural society has a tendency to be closely connected with the earth, to be sedentary and unified. On the other hand, the cattle-raising society is less sedentary and moves around freely like animals. It is active and innovative and has a tendency toward acquisition. Eastern cultures, with their roots in the earth like plants and their strong tendency toward the pursuit of a fundamental world within the internal self, are yin cultures. Epoch-making Western cultures, which are active like animals, trying to possess the outside world, are yang cultures. It may be said that the theory of yin and yang stated in these terms reveals the advantages and disadvantages of Eastern and Western cultures, not unlike those of their respective medicines. The East—particularly India, where there is a strong tendency to see matter as *maya* (illusion) —culturally overestimates spirituality and, after having been defeated by modern war policies, has come under the control of the various Western colonial powers. On the other hand, Western material civilization, bent on global domination, is inviting an environmental crisis by exploiting nature without consideration of the planet as a whole.

Yin Culture	Yang Culture
Eastern medicine	Western medicine
natural	artificial
philosophical	scientific
plants	animals
maternal qualities	paternal qualities
passive	active
holistic	divisional
unconscious	conscious
intuitive	analytical
union of mind and body	duality of mind and body

The Eastern View of Life

The Part and the Whole

Western medicine understands life analytically and the body as a collection of organs not unlike the different parts of a machine. This is because it is founded on natural science, which is based on Descartes's theory of the duality of the mind and body. Natural science is a discipline that isolates the individual's subjectivity (the mind) from objective nature (matter). It is the study of nature by reduction of the "whole" to individual constituents. In the West this methodology has also been applied to medical treatment, which has come to see the mind and body as separate entities, disregarding the mind and treating the body as matter.

Since each organ of the body is seen as having its own individual existence, illness is diagnosed as an abnormality of one part of the body and the mutual relationship between the respective organs is not considered. This analytical view of life is at present generally more accepted than the holistic view offered by Oriental medicine. Therefore, when people become ill, they visit the hospital without considering that the cause of their illness may be a disorder in the whole body, an imbalance between the mind and body, or problems in lifestyle. Once in the hospital, to answer the patient's questions of "What is wrong with me?" the doctor performs a detailed analysis using x-rays and other examination equipment and reports, for instance, "You have a bad liver." Then the doctor attempts to cure the illness as though carrying out repairs on a broken machine. The problem with this approach to medical treatment is that the illness is confined to one part of the body without taking into consideration the possibility that the patient may have in fact created the illness. Oriental medicine considers the symptoms to be a reflection of disorder in the whole body. In other words, the symptoms in one part of the body are the local manifestations of the burden of an overall disorder in the patient's energy. If the part of the body showing symptoms of malfunction is surgically removed, the disorder will seek to manifest itself elsewhere in the body. This type of manifestation is evident in patients who repeatedly undergo surgical operations.

According to Shizuto Masunaga,[7] because illness results from the patient's way of life, the search for the cause of the illness allows the patient to reflect upon his or her lifestyle. Whatever the cause may be, the doctor's fundamental obligation is aiding the patient's self-discovery. In a shiatsu clinic, for example, through treatment, patients learn to communicate with their inner nature.

Western medicine has long carried out treatment with disregard to the patient's mind. However, in recent years, with the development of psychosomatic medicine, psychotherapy has been attempted on patients with physical ailments. Psychosomatic medicine claims that patients who repeatedly undergo surgical operations for gastric ulcers, for example, have psychological causes underlying the ailment and should be treated accordingly. However, even if psychosomatic medicine were to become the medicine of

---

7.   Shizuto Masunaga (1925–1981), born in Hiroshima in a family of shiatsu practitioners, began practicing shiatsu in the late 1940s. He discovered the twelve meridians throughout the body from the six-meridian system noted in the Classics and developed the system of meridianal diagnosis.

the future for everyone, it is still based on natural science and has the inherent weakness of being unable to surpass the theory of the duality of the mind and body. Therefore, when the results of therapy are not immediately visible on the patient's body, even where attention is focused on the mind, Western medicine fails because it has, in fact, no ideology or technique equipped to heal both the mind and body as one entity. It is believed that this is because the West lacks insight into the fundamental concept of *ki*.

To understand the true medical significance of the union of the mind and body, one must recognize the existence of energy channels, known as *meridians*, throughout the body. Through the application of technological science, Western medicine has reached a detailed understanding of the different elements that make up the human body. However, this excludes the holistic method of perceiving life as the union of the mind and body. In the Eastern view, life is considered "organic; each part works in coordination with the whole"; and "continuous and successive; life continues and one form succeeds another." First of all, the view that life is organically coordinated means that all life exists as one, and each part of the whole has a mutually coordinated interrelationship. Second, the view that life is continuous and successive means that each individual life does not exist apart from all other life but has a continuous and coordinated organic link with everything in nature.

One characteristic of the Eastern view is that life is perceived to be an exchange of energy rather than an accumulation of matter. Therefore, each part that makes up the whole does not exist individually but has a mutually organic interrelationship and its existence is linked with the existence of every other part. It may be said that in Eastern thought this is where the interrelationship between the part and the whole is most evident. Unlike natural science, Eastern ideology holds that the whole is more important than the sum total of the parts it constitutes. In Buddhism this is expressed as "one in all and all in one," which is a fundamental belief that the whole universe is reflected in even one speck of dust.

Oriental medicine sees the whole body as one small universe. This is because it is founded on the relationship between the whole (creation) and the part (the body), and on the Theory of the Five Elements of Yin and Yang, which claims that the same energy circulating in creation also circulates within the human body. Eastern ideology further claims that "the whole is the part and the part is the whole." The fact that life is understood as energy and not as a physical composition means that the essence of life and nature is a state of continuous and relentless change rather than stagnant matter. If one were to take a spinning top as an example of life, natural science of the West would focus on the structure of the object, while Oriental medicine would focus on its vigorous rotation. The perception of nature in Eastern philosophy is that everything is in constant flow and change and that the essence of life is not to be found in a fixed moment but in change; for fixation means death. The essence of life means that the whole exists as a whole and cannot be separated or isolated from everything else. Furthermore, everything is made up of everything else, and physical bodies in the natural world are vessels for the circulation of energy.

Because Oriental medicine perceives the cause of illness to be in the holistic nature of life, the aim is to establish harmony between nature and the patient; in other words, "the whole and the part." In Oriental medicine, it is believed that the energy of creation circulates through the body, and the meridians are the vessels that carry this energy throughout the body. Therefore all physical and biological functions and psychological phenomena appear through the action of the meridians. For example, shiatsu therapy to the Large Intestine Meridian can physically cure a skin disease and a sore throat and simultaneously heighten the psychological power of expression in the patient. Because meridians determine psychological phenomena and physiological functions, Tao shiatsu heals within the union of the mind and body, and the holistic nature of life can be better understood and personally experienced through treatment in the shiatsu clinic.

Reductionism and Health

As previously mentioned, the Eastern view of life is not shared by everyone. This is perhaps because it is not well known. Many patients are surprised when in shiatsu therapy, their neck pain is relieved by pressure to a meridian in the leg and wonder how the two parts of the body may be connected. This shows the extent to which the reductionist view of isolating all parts of the body is generally accepted, and how little is known about the holistic view of the body.

In modern times natural science, based on reductionism, has been accepted as the only truth. People have faith in the scientific technology that allows them to live in materialistic luxury, thinking that science and technology can and will solve all problems, and progress in medicine will cure all disease. But is this really so? Although highly precise technological equipment has been developed, new drugs are continually released, and the number of hospitals has increased, the number of patients and sick people is not actually decreasing. In fact, the effect is the opposite; each year the money spent on health care continues to increase. In Japan for instance, the rate of increase in health care spending exceeds the rate of economic growth. In America, despite the fact that health care costs are 10 percent of the GNP, or one and a half times the national defense budget, the number of people being treated for illness continues to grow.

There are many reasons for this. First, living in developed, materialist countries creates psychological and physical stress. Second, industrial waste pollutes and destroys the environment, which in turn affects our health through the air we breathe, the water we drink, and the soil that provides our food. Also, because of modern farming methods, very little of the food we eat is natural. Prior to industrialization, people ate food that was grown organically according to the cycles of nature and fertilized with human and domestic animal excrement. Modern farming ignores the cycles of nature, and through the use of chemical fertilizers over the years, the soil becomes barren and food grown there lacks not only taste but also valuable nutrients essential for the health of humankind.

Western scientists analyze the elements such as phosphorous and potassium that make up natural fertilizers and artificially manufacture chemical fertilizers with the same compounds. This too is indicative of the reductionist perspective, which maintains that a compound similar to one that occurs naturally can be made artificially, simply by analyzing the elements that make up the whole. It does not acknowledge that fertilizer may be one energy that makes up part of the collective whole. The use of artificial fertilizers and agricultural chemicals renders the earth infertile and pollutes the environment. Modern farming disregards nature's cycles and ignores the condition of the soil because it can only see as far as the next harvest. People pay for this mistake with their own health. Some Japanese doctors, surprised at the number of illnesses caused by agricultural chemicals, have formed their own farming communities to integrate medicine and farming.

The reductionist perspective influences the modern diet in other ways as well. For example, most of the foods people consume are either refined or have artificial additives. Refined foods such as white rice, white bread, white sugar, and chemical salts are deficient in natural vitamins and minerals.

Modern nutritionists, conforming to the principles of reductionism, advise that vitamins and minerals lost in the process of refining foods may be supplemented by eating other foods. This is because food too is understood as a compound of elements divisible by chemical equation and not as the energy that nurtures life. However, it is better to take a balance of nutritious elements from whole foods than to try to create a balance by taking each individually, because unless all nutritious elements such as proteins and carbohydrates are taken together, they are not absorbed. Furthermore, an intake of white sugar, artificial flavors, and food additives depletes the body of vitamins, minerals, calcium, and so on, which cannot always be supplemented by other foods.

Realizing the Holistic Nature of Life

In ancient times in the East, the body was thought to be "the shrine of the spirit" where the power of nature dwelled. In modern times, because the materialist civilization relies on natural science, elemental reductionism has permeated all aspects of society, and the body is seen as nothing more than one element contributing to social productivity. (This ideology is also apparent in the modern marriage where a partner is reduced to a combination of such classifications as income, position and character, and so on.)

People surround themselves with electrical appliances for comfort and convenience, continuing to ignore the serious negative aspects that accompany this lifestyle. Even after the end of the Cold War, the manufacturing of weapons continues, and there are already enough nuclear bombs in the world to destroy the planet many times over, creating subconscious, if not conscious, anxiety in everyone. Furthermore, when the environment is manipulated to suit people's immediate needs, the cycles of nature are damaged and environmental pollution from industrial waste increases.

The controlled modern urban lifestyle, with its pervasive dependence on cars and electrical appliances, hinders the natural intimate rapport between people. It fosters isolation and a loss of the true essence of life. Recently, people have attempted to regain the true experience of life by becoming enthusiastic about sports and by trying to enhance their sexual lives. "Rational thought," which relies on the function of the forebrain, is essential for life in the modern world, but excessive activity of the forebrain suppresses the function of the midbrain, which is responsible for emotions and instincts (chapter 1). When the activity of the midbrain is suppressed, it becomes difficult for people to express themselves and to experience life fully. This suppression of the midbrain may explain the depression and discordance suffered by many city dwellers.

The most practical aspect of shiatsu is the projection of the true sensation of life onto the patient. This may be one of the principal reasons for the popularity of shiatsu in modern times. To experience the true sensation of life means to actually feel its holistic nature, which can only take place when harmony with nature is established. The aim of all Oriental medicine, not just shiatsu therapy, is to restore the patient's harmony with nature. Therefore, Oriental medicine, unlike Western medicine, does not diagnose an illness by identifying its name through the classifications of particular symptoms. It looks at the condition of harmony with nature and carries out *sho diagnosis* (chapter 4), which forecasts a pattern in the healing response.

The patient's degree of harmony with nature cannot be measured with examination equipment. When people are in harmony with nature, the energy of *ki* exists in them and in nature equally. However, because *ki* is not comparable to anything that may be measured quantitatively, there is no way to recognize harmony with nature and *ki* without perceiving the patient's feelings. The *ki* energy of creation exists in all dimensions. When *ki* in the patient's body and mind is in excess, the patient is diagnosed as *jitsu*, and when it is deficient, he or she is diagnosed as *kyo* (chapter 3). Because the *ki* energy of nature cannot be expressed quantitatively, a condition cannot be diagnosed as *kyo* or *jitsu* by mechanical methods. It is the disharmony with nature created by the tenacity of the ego that generates the disorders in energy known as *kyo* and *jitsu*.

Oriental diagnosis begins with what is known as *boshin*—general diagnosis through looking at the whole (chapter 5). In the Classics, *boshin*, which identifies five different colors on the patient's face, is described as a method of diagnosis. However, I believe *boshin* essentially means the union of the healer with nature and the actual sensation of the state of harmony between the patient and nature. When the healer actually feels the patient's vitality as though it were his or her own, both the patient and healer become one with nature. In other words, when healers surpass the distinction of "you and I," they are able to unite with the vitality of nature, which enables them to respond to even the most subtle feelings of disquiet within their patients. It is at this point that they are able to sense their patients' vitality as their own. In Oriental medicine, diagnosis is carried out in conjunction with this response to vital energy. The reason Oriental medicine does not use examination equipment in diagnosis, then, is not that it lags behind modern times but that intangible life and the feeling of oneness with nature cannot be determined by sophisticated examination equipment. Also, because meridians do not exist as anatomically discernible parts of the body, correct diagnosis in the Eastern sense cannot be performed through the use of machinery.

The concept of meridians was first developed by the ancient Chinese through Taoist disciplines known as *sendo* (chapter 1) and the practice of breathing techniques, not by the Western method of research through autopsy. In the East, research is performed through intuition and through personal experience that surpasses analysis and intellectualization. On the other hand, Western research is analytical and rational thought is applied intellectually. Meridians can be felt only through personal experience and therefore belong to a world indefinable by words. Clinically, the position and depth of meridians varies infinitely according to each person. If healers are not capable of responding to this infinite variety, they are not able to identify and affect the meridians correctly. When healers understand everything as "the work of life," through an understanding of the meridians, they are also able to realize the infinite power of continuous change that pervades existence. Furthermore, they are able to understand that an individual's existence has an indivisible relationship with everything and cannot be isolated from the rest of creation.

Through the study of meridians we understand the essence of life as the union of the objective and the subjective. As explained above, meridians cannot be analyzed objectively or perceived intellectually. The only way to understand meridians, and therefore life, is through the holistic response of the patient's vital energies stimulated by the healer. In modern times too much emphasis has been placed on rational thought, and the worldview put forward by natural science of the West has all too readily been accepted as the only truth. We have reached an era where we must be liberated from the perception that the one and only absolute truth is that which can be "proved" analytically.

Students who take courses in shiatsu are led to an understanding that enables them to feel these cultural differences between the East and West. Japanese students have a tendency to carry out what their teacher tells them without question or doubt. But Western students seek theoretical foundation for what they are told. Japanese students follow their teacher silently, but Western students want first of all to know *why*. Each of these methods of approach to knowledge has merits and demerits. If the whole world were like the former, it would lack the strength to surpass tradition and generate innovations, while if it were like the latter, there would be no understanding of concepts that surpass verbal definition, such as the essence of Eastern culture.

The Role of Tao Shiatsu
in the Twenty-First Century

Understanding Meridians

Based on natural science, and in particular on the view of the world proposed by physics, Western medicine has until now carried out specific treatment on each affected area of the body. However, life cannot be analyzed by its elemental composition, and the view of nature pervasive in the East since ancient times, beginning to be emphasized in the West, is that of the existence of mutual interrelationships. It is essential that from now on, the true state of illness be diagnosed from the point of view of the holistic nature of life and the interrelationship of the mind and body rather than treated as an abnormality of a specific organ.

The book *Health and Healing* by Andrew Weil proposes that the future goal of medicine should be the perfectly mutual exchange between the mind and the body.[8] This leads to the understanding that the significance of studying meridians is to provide clinical proof of the "oneness" of the mind and the body.

Meridians were discovered as a means of cure based on treatment through sympathy between the patient and doctor. In fact, meridians cannot be un-

---

8.   Andrew Weil, *Health and Healing: Understanding Conventional and Alternative Medicine* (Boston: Houghton Mifflin, 1983).

derstood outside the concept and practice of curing the patient through touch of the skin (the manual techniques of shiatsu). Recent attempts to scientifically prove the existence of meridians by electrical responses in the living body have not succeeded because what can be scientifically proven is limited to the quantitative expressions of scientific method. For example, the scientific analysis of light cannot go beyond quantitative expressions of wavelength and wave form. However, for the human eye, light is color. Color is qualitative; in other words, it belongs in the realm of people's actual sensitivity and subjectivity.[9] Anything closely connected to the true essence of life cannot be expressed quantitatively because its nature is qualitative, comprising actual sensations such as pleasantness or unpleasantness. It is also possible to say that the true essence of life exists in the qualitative nature of meridians. (In much the same way, the existence of black holes and quarks is merely inferred and the physicist Sharron notes that these belong in the realm of the unobservable void of existence.)

Because of their qualitative nature, meridians can only be perceived by an equally qualitative human mind. Healers are able to recognize meridians when they are in sympathy with the patient's vital energies and there is a fusion between the feelings of the two. The union of the healer's mind with that of the patient means that the former is in tune with the latter's vitality. Scientific analysis, on the other hand, is carried out by the mind, which distinguishes between the self and others without any preconception of this union.

Some maintain that it is inconceivable to feel another's life sensations as one's own. The essence of life is something that we are all able to experience in daily life. It derives from a common source; for instance, when we are with healthy people we also begin to become healthy. In some African tribes, when a woman gives birth, her husband screams in agony, seemingly experiencing the pain of childbirth, and as a result, the woman appears to feel no pain at all. We all have the potential to feel a mutual sympathy with others because all living things belong to one fundamental universality. By being in sympathy with the patient's vitality, the healer can become one with the source of life, and in so doing, the healer is able to feel the other person's life as his or her own. It is through this that meridians are recognized and understood.

---

9. Mitsuo Ishikawa, *Toyoteki Seimeikan to Gakumon* [in Japanese] (Tokyo: Sanshintosho Publishers, 1983).

Release of Lymbic System through Shiatsu

In materialist cultures, people's lives are focused on discrimination and rationalization—functions carried out by the forebrain. Increased forebrain activity increases conscious action of the ego and inhibits the function of the lymbic system of the midbrain. This weakens the ability to empathize with the lives of others and the ability to actually feel the strength and vitality of life energies.

Urban dwellers are often said to be "cold." It is thought that living in cities actually weakens primitive consciousness as it weakens people's ability to sympathize with and respond to others. Many city dwellers suffer from the so-called midbrain syndrome, an imbalance in the autonomic nervous system caused by the suppression of instincts and of the activity of the lymbic system (see Figure I.3). The lymbic system is the storage place of all memories of the past and all the idiosyncrasies created by one's external experiences and childhood. Because of this, the lymbic system is known as the seat of the subconscious self. Stress, fear, and anxiety distort the lymbic system, suppress the autonomic nervous functions and internal secretion, and reduce immunity to illness. Therefore, as much as patients are said to be ailing physically, the psychological burdens from their past and stress created by their social environment are very closely linked with their condition.

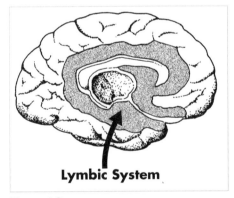

Lymbic System

Figure I.3

If we are to attain spiritual peace and heighten our bodies' homeostasis, we must be liberated from the excess activity of the forebrain and activate the functions of the lymbic system. As well as being responsible for instinctive action and emotions, the lymbic system is deeply connected with the autonomic nerves. Eastern meditation and the various methods of maintaining one's health, such as yoga and martial arts, have begun to attract attention as means of promoting general well-being because they are believed to heal distortion in the lymbic system.

The lymbic system is directly influenced by touch on the skin. Therefore, the steady, constant pressure of shiatsu, while relaxing the patient and enhancing responses, also releases disorders in this part of the brain. Nervous tensions are manifested as muscular tension, but the relaxation of the skin of the entire body brought about by shiatsu causes a catharsis and relaxation in the subconscious. One effect of shiatsu therapy is helping patients gain insight into the subconscious cause of their suffering. Through therapy on meridians, patients are urged to face their problems without the intervention of words. Furthermore, the healing process of Tao shiatsu purifies the patient's subconscious and encourages spiritual growth.

Chapter One

Ki and Shiatsu Healing Techniques

What Is *Ki?*

The Meaning of *Ki*

The Oriental concept of *ki* is very difficult to define. In China, the word *ki* originally expressed the tangible significance of vital energy. In Japan, the word has been in daily use throughout the centuries since the infiltration of Chinese culture first began. *Ki* expresses the concept of the fundamental energies of the universe, of which nature and the functions of the human mind and body are a part.

In Japanese the word *ki* combines with other words to form phrases used to describe natural, supernatural, physical, and psychological phenomena. For example, the Japanese word for weather is *ten-ki* (the *ki* of heaven), atmospheric pressure is *ki-atsu* (the pressure of *ki*), and air is *ku-ki* (the *ki* of the sky). *Ki* appears in phrases that express psychological sensitivity such as "it feels good," *ki-mochi ga yoi* (to have/hold "good" *ki*). The phrase *ki ga chiru* (to scatter one's *ki*) describes the inability to focus one's mind. (Chuang-tsu used this phrase to mean "one's death.") The word *ki* is also used in daily expressions such as "How are you?" *genki desuka* (*gen-ki* is the source of universal energy, so this greeting asks, "Are you filled with universal energy?"). The character 気 (*ki* or *ke*) also describes occult phenomena, as in the expression *mono no ke* (a supernatural being).

There are also many phrases in the Japanese language that use the word *ki* to express the psychology of a person. These phrases indicate that the psychology of living things is determined by the type of *ki* in and around them. For instance, asking someone what kind of *ki* another person or thing has is in fact asking what sort of impression he or she has of that person or thing. If the person projects a positive image, one says *ki-mochi ga yoi* (he or she has "good *ki*"). When one likes someone or something, the phrase *ki ni iru* (to enter one's *ki*) is used, meaning that the *ki* of that person or thing flows freely into oneself. If two people have a good relationship, it is said that they each suit the other's *ki, ki ga au. Ki ga aru* means that there is love between two people, for it says that *ki* is present between them. The phrases *ki ni suru, ki gakari,* and *ki ni naru* all express the human psychological phenomena of anxiety. *Ki* is also used to express people's character: for example, a person who has a short temper is a person with short *ki* (*ki ga mijikai*), whereas a relaxed person is someone who has extensive *ki* (*ki ga nagai*). As illustrated by these examples, *ki* is commonly used in daily Japanese to describe the energy in nature and in the various psychological aspects of the human mind and body.

In ancient China, because *ki* was the force that initiated all physical and psychological functions, the concept held a place in medicine, the martial arts, sorcery, and many other aspects of life. Initially used for military purposes, *ki* divination is said to have begun with determining when soldiers' strength was at its highest, according to which the army appropriated military movement. Following this, the study of *ki* developed into a practical way of predicting people's destiny through the ability of the diviner to judge or read a person's *ki.*

One ancient Chinese discipline for maintaining one's health and well-being that used the fundamental concept of *ki* is *sendo. Sendo,* forms of which are still practiced today, has two types of therapies: *nai-tan,* an internal drug produced by the body, and *gai-tan,*[1] an external drug produced outside the body and ingested. *Gai-tan* resembles alchemy, in which the elixir of immortality is created and ingested. The original form of *sendo* is believed to be based on *nai-tan,* meaning that the elixir of immortality is produced internally by the body, through self-discipline.

In *sendo,* yang *ki* energy is generated in the body by means of a breathing technique originally known as *busoku.*[2] This discipline causes yang to ascend the Governor Vessel in the inner spinal column, pass through the *hyakue* point at the center of the top of the head, descend through the front of the body via the Conception Vessel, and collect at a point in the lower abdomen called the *tanden* (see Figure 1.1). In *sendo,* yang *ki* energy is said to circulate through the Governor and Conception Vessels by the microcosmic circuit and, in a particular sequence, through meridians throughout the body

---

1. *Tan* pill, elixir, and so on. Appears in words such as *sentan,* the elixir (of life). *Gai,* external, outside. *Nai,* internal, inside.
2. *Busoku,* martial arts breathing technique. *Bu* means military art or glory; *soku* means breath. *Busoku* literally means "the breath of the warrior."

by the macrocosmic circuit. This circulation of yang *ki* energy is a fundamental aspect of the disciplines of *sendo*. When this process takes place, the elixir of eternal life is secreted in a person's saliva. The points of the Conception Vessel closely resemble the yoga chakras. Similarly, the mystical experience of yang *ki* energy passing through the Conception Vessel may be likened to Kundalini yoga. These similarities may indicate that *sendo* is a synthesis of the Chinese idea of meridians and the Indian practice of yoga.

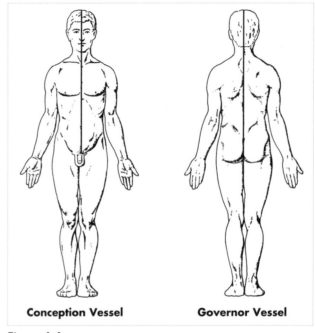

Conception Vessel   **Governor Vessel**

Figure 1.1

The practice of Eastern disciplines heightens the sensitivity and movement of *ki* and enables the mind and body to become one. Practicing these disciplines, one gains the profound realization that *ki* exists as the source of everything. Originally, the ultimate purpose of *sendo* was the attainment of immortality; however, today its disciplines are put to more practical uses, such as the enhancement of health and the healing of illness. A good example of one aspect of the discipline presently practiced throughout China is *qigong*, which has been proven effective by scientific study and is valued as a significant method of maintaining one's health and well-being.

Other disciplines, such as the martial arts that originated in the East, have adopted the basic concept of *ki* and aim to achieve infinite strength through its integration. One of the basic techniques of Chinese martial arts is blocking the opponent's *ki* by hindering its flow through the meridians. Experts such as Aoki, the founder of Shintaido, use another method, the *toate* technique,[3] to throw the opponent to the ground using the force of *ki* without any actual physical contact whatsoever. There are many masters in martial arts who have this ability, one of whom is Master Morihei Ueshiba, founder of aikido. In one of the many well-known stories about Master Ueshiba, a famous Japanese baseball player was, when he met Ueshiba, told to take hold of the master's wooden sword as though it were a baseball bat and hit Ueshiba with it. The moment the baseball player did this, he lost consciousness. When he regained consciousness he found himself lying on the ground with no recollection of having fallen. In another story, Ueshiba asked a karate master to attack him from any angle. When he kicked Ueshiba, the karate master fell to the ground without knowing how it happened. In all such stories, Ueshiba used his ability to manipulate *ki* freely by unifying with it. It is worth noting that Ueshiba was believed to be over seventy years old when both these incidents took place.

The concept of *ki,* supported amply by actual physical experiences such as those described above, is fundamental to Chinese philosophy and culture. Through an awareness of its existence and through personal experience, the ancient Chinese recognized methods of developing *ki* through disciplinary techniques of the mind and body. In the East there was a strong tendency toward the empirical rather than the intellectual understanding of life. Perhaps this is why both yoga and Zen meditation strive toward spiritual enlightenment, placing great emphasis on physical postures and breathing techniques. In Tantric Buddhism, it is said that hand gestures called mudra lead a person to enlightenment. Similarly, beating the wooden block when chanting Buddhist mantras is thought to lead to enlightenment. A particular characteristic of Eastern religions is the attempt to transmit the body itself into enlightenment. Therefore, when Dogen, the founder of a Japanese Zen Buddhist sect, is asked, "Is it the mind or the body that becomes enlightened?" he replies, "It is both the mind and body."

The East has long recognized that the body and the mind do not exist as separate entities. Therefore all aspects of Eastern culture (philosophy, art,

---

3. *To-ate,* a martial arts technique. Characters suggest "striking or aiming from afar." A technique where the power of *ki* is used to strike down the opponent without actual physical touch.

martial arts, medicine, and so on) strive to attain freedom in universal life through an empirical understanding of the fundamental union of the mind and body. *Ki* unifies the very basis of the mind and body and at the same time has a mutual relationship with all things at the source of creation. All living things result from the power of *ki*, which is said to fill the universe, nurture the whole of creation by its pervasive presence, and at the same time exist as "one." Lyle Watson's famous story of One Hundred Monkeys begins with one monkey on a particular island starting to wash potatoes in the sea. Before long, this habit spread to other monkeys throughout the island, and soon even monkeys on other islands started to wash their potatoes in the sea before eating them. This may be taken as an illustration of the existence of *ki* as one at the source of all life.

The cultural system that emerged in China, with its profound respect for the practical application of theories and concepts, was almost totally founded on the basis of the actual experience of *ki*. It saw the birth and application of *ki* in medicine, methods of maintaining and enhancing physical and psychological health and well-being, the martial arts, divination, and the ways of searching for immortality practiced in *sendo*.

Ki: The Unifier of Mind and Matter

The I Ching preaches that "all things in creation are born and nurtured by the union of yin and yang." This means that the mutually complementary and reciprocal polarities known as yin and yang, which exist as one in their essence, generate all the manifestations in nature. The source where yin and yang exist together as one is called *Tao*, and *ki* is the energy that initiates the force of manifestations and vicissitudes of these two polarities. The I Ching explains the importance of the harmony of yin and yang and states that the condition of *ki* is determined by changes in the balance of these two polarities. The imbalance of yin and yang not only influences the fate and well-being of the individual but also is manifested in society as a whole, causing disturbances and natural disasters throughout the world.

The individual's *ki* and the *ki* of nature are inextricably bound and mutually influenced. For instance, when we say that a day of fine weather brightens the heart, it is because our *ki* functions in sympathy with the *ki* of nature, which in turn is in sympathy with each and every person in the world. Similarly, it is said that excessive negativity existing among a people contributes to the causes of natural disasters. During the latter part of this century, predictions, warnings, and occurrences of natural disasters have increased all over the world. It could be said that this phenomenon is directly attributable to disorders in people's *ki.*

When the mind and body are perceived as a duality (as in the West), it is difficult to accept the concept that mind and matter are born from the same *ki.* For example, some Western brain surgeons maintain that the mind is nothing but the physical structure of the matter that makes up the brain, which functions merely through electrochemical reactions. Recently, however, in the field of medicine, the ideology of the mind-body dichotomy has begun to diminish. This has been mostly attributable to discoveries about the placebo effect, where a placebo (or "fake" drug) is used to alleviate pain or to actually cure a specific ailment. In one experiment, patients complaining of headaches were given a placebo made of wheat flour, having been told it was a headache cure. The results showed that a high ratio of patients experienced pain relief. This is because, by suggestion, the pain-relieving substance endorphin (which is a morphine) is released by the brain. If the patient whose pain has been relieved by the placebo effect is then given a drug to suppress the release of endorphin in the brain, the pain returns. This shows that the placebo effect takes place when the release of endorphin is stimulated through suggestion. In view of such findings, it is important to note that the former saying of pragmatic science "mind does not influence matter" cannot hold true.

The unification of mind and matter can also be understood from the perspective of Einstein's formula of the theory of general relativity, $E = MC^2$ (energy equals mass multiplied by the square of the speed of light), which indicates that matter and energy are interchangeable. The atomic bomb, for instance, creates destructive power by changing matter into energy. If matter is energy and we think of the mind as also being energy, matter and the structure of the mind can be described as two forms of energy, just as ice and vapor are two forms of water. Buddhism also describes mind and matter as different forms of one and the same energy. The Buddhist sutras mention that coarse energy vibrations represent physical energy while subtle vibrations represent spiritual energy. Matter is known as an objective idea while the mind is a subjective one, but at their source they are one; both are recognized as the absolute Buddha nature. This is known as the great spirit of the universe, or Amitâvha.

Ki is not a tangible substance, but through Eastern disciplines the mind's eye can be opened to it and its presence can be clearly felt. Many Eastern cultures are based upon this notion. However, for Westerners, *ki* is a relatively new concept, and since there is a strong tendency to intellectualize everything in terms of scientific and cultural analysis, the concept of *ki*, which is difficult to explain either linguistically or quantitatively, is not easily understood.

In 1984, with East-West cultural exchange as its aim, a conference entitled "Technological Science and the Spiritual World" was held in Japan. Japanese scholars and martial arts masters presented research papers on *ki* and gave demonstrations. However, many Western academics were not convinced of the existence of *ki*. In the newspapers, a philosophy of science professor from Harvard University was reported as saying that it was extremely difficult to solve the riddle of *ki* energy and asking if *ki* had a direction and if it could be revived. Also, a professor in molecular biology asked, "What on earth is *ki*? Can its existence be proven? The Japanese seem to have a good understanding of *ki*, but is there a way for Westerners, who have a different cultural background, to understand it also?"[4]

An understanding of the concept of *ki* is fundamental to an understanding of Japanese culture. The Japanese themselves need little explanation that *ki*, although unanalyzable, is a pervasive and vital force. However, there is no such cultural background in the West and no suitable word or concept to express *ki*. Besides, religious judgment has existed throughout Western history and for a long time science was restrained by the doctrines of the church. There was, therefore, a strong tendency to reject as unscientific or untrue those things that could not be explained logically or did not fit established preconceptions.

Ki is difficult to define within a Western framework because it is said to be based on direct experience and not on actual fact that may be expressed quantitatively or linguistically. At the conference the contrary opinions on *ki* indicated in the discussions between Western and Eastern academics demonstrate the difficulty of reaching a mutual understanding between people of fundamentally different cultural backgrounds and histories. However, the

---

4. Mitsuo Ishikawa, *Nyu Saiensu no Sekaikan* [in Japanese] (Tokyo: Tama, 1985).

fact that this discussion took place at all may suggest that the curtain to a new era has opened.

Classification of Energy: *Shin, Ki,* and *Sei*

Life functions are performed by the energy of the universe within the individual and the three types of energy—*shin, ki,* and *sei*—into which it changes. *Shin* (god, deity, mind, soul) is mental and spiritual energy, and *ki* is the motive force of vital functions. *Sei* (spirit, vitality, energy, excellence, purity) energy, which may be explained as the essence of *ki,* is the embodiment of sexual energy. *Shin, ki,* and *sei* are at the same time innate and acquired. *Shin* energy (also known as *shikishin*) determines conscious action. The functions of cognition are carried out by the transformation of *ki* into *shin.* Linguistically in Japanese, the character *shin* means the mind as well as the soul and appears in words such as *shisshin* (to lose consciousness), and *seishin* (the essence of the spirit). Innate *shin* signifies the unconscious, while acquired *shin* refers to actual consciousness. *Shin* corresponds to the Heart Meridian.

Innate *ki* is supposed to be present from the beginning of life in the fetus, while acquired *ki* is said to accumulate externally after birth. There are three types of acquired *ki* energy: *ten no ki,* which is known as "*ki* of the breath" and exists as air; *chi-ki* (also called "*ki* of the earth"), which is *ki* that rises from the earth and materializes as water and food; and *meridianal ki,* which is said to be the foundation of all life activity. *Ki* is said to flow through the Kidney Meridian first. This is why in Eastern martial arts the most important energy point in the body is the point below the navel that corresponds to the Kidney Meridian; it is understood to be the center of *ki.*

Sei energy is the essence of *ki* and appears in the Japanese word *seizui,* meaning essence. *Sei* is related to reproductive activity and is the initial motive force of action. Innate *sei* is said to be the unformed energy of vitality and action, whereas acquired *sei* has tangible form, such as semen. According to Taoism, boys are active and energetic because they do not discharge acquired *sei* through semen, and it is thought that if adult men were as active as boys they would not survive very long. The aim of Taoist training is to heighten the vital force to the level of that of a child by transforming *sei* into *ki* (i.e. the transformation of sexual energy).[5]

Literary records claim that Taoism was transmitted through the ages to the emperors of ancient China by a god called Tenshi Tenson (T'ien-Shih T'ien-Tsun in Chinese), and it is said to have been transmitted to Lao-Tzu by the legendary Yellow Emperor. Since the oldest medical classic of the East, *The Yellow Emperor's Classic of Internal Medicine*, also derives from the Yellow Emperor, it is clear that Taoism and Oriental medicine are closely linked. The three classifications of energy, *shin*, *ki*, and *sei*, are noted in *The Yellow Emperor's Classic of Internal Medicine*. However, although these classifications are said to play a significant role in the principles of Taoism, they do not appear to have held any importance in acupuncture. Furthermore, Taoism further developed into *doin* and *ankyo*, which are generally known as *shinsen-jutsu* (the art of immortality; *"shin"* here is the same word defined above) and played a significant role in the development of manual Oriental medicine, or "Tao Shiatsu," as we know it today.

Ki and Image

The Power of "Image" in Therapy

Ki unifies the mind and body, integrating the conscious and the unconscious. The omnipresent *ki* in the universe complies with and responds to certain mental images, generating bodily functions and psychological phenomena. Therefore, the influence of *ki* on the functions of the mind and body depends on the image of the outside world held by each individual. An inherent human characteristic is the belief that we live through our own volition; however, our lives are actually maintained through images and an intimate rapport with the *ki* of the external world.

The concept that *ki* complies with images can be supported by demonstrations designed by the Ki Society (*Ki no Kenkyukai*), which set out to prove

---

5. Because of this theoretical background, the Art of Love-Making, a training technique of the mind and body used to heighten the vital forces through sex, played an important role in the Chinese Classics and was seriously studied in ancient China.

the notion that the mind and body do not exist as separate entities. For example, if a person is told to touch his forehead with the palms of his hands and to hold in his mind an image of not letting go under any circumstances, a second person who is asked to try and pull the first person's hands away from his forehead will be unable to do so. In another experiment, if someone is told to extend his arm and imagine water flowing down his arm and through his hand, another person when asked is unable to bend the extended arm. Such experiments help us to understand certain aspects of the mystery of the power of *ki* and the potential effects of mental images on one's body. When the omnipresent *ki* of the universe is visualized, people are able to draw on untapped strength. (This is what happens when people faced with extreme danger can perform extraordinary feats.[6]) The power of *ki*, however, is by no means limited to incidents of danger. All actions of our mind and body in daily life are performed through *ki*, whose essence and direction are in turn determined by mental images.

A more pertinent example of the way in which *ki* functions through visualization is the mystery of the famous Lourdes Springs in Europe, where invalids immerse themselves in the waters of the natural spring to regain the ability to walk. More than the known elements in the waters of the spring, such as germanium, it is the expectations and beliefs of the patients, who are told that they can expect to be cured by the spring, that play a major role in the healing process. In fact, because the patients undoubtedly already have a distinct image of their own cured body as they prepare to go to the spring, many improve even before arriving in Lourdes. It is thought that *ki* works by complying with such images of cures for illness and disease. Because of *ki*'s response to images, the importance of visualization has begun to attract the attention of people involved in various methods of physical training. For instance, ski-jump competitors, sprint athletes, racers, and other Olympic athletes strive to visualize themselves as winners even before competition begins. Once they have formed this image, they are capable of achieving excellent results.

---

6. *Kajiba no bakajikara* is a Japanese phrase for the almost supernatural strength a person is able to summon in times of extreme danger. There is no English equivalent for this phrase. It roughly translates to "one's absurd strength when one's house is on fire," and implies that such strength is brought about by *ki*.

Visualization is also used in the Simonton method of cancer therapy, which achieves successful results by suggesting an image of dying cancer cells to the patient. A visualization technique known as the *nanso* method has been in use in Japan since ancient times. This healing practice is said to have been taught to the famous Zen priest Hakuin by a sage when, during his youth, he became ill from overpracticing the disciplines. Explained in simple terms, this healing method uses the image of a warm, healing liquid being circulated throughout the body from the head. Unfortunately, the true significance of a healing method that works through this type of visualization is not generally understood by medical practitioners. Nonetheless, it is of utmost importance for understanding the mutual relationship between mind and body. One example that demonstrates this importance is the placebo effect mentioned earlier. The placebo, a drug without any medicinal properties whatsoever, has the potential to cure an ailment because, through suggestion, it causes endorphin to be secreted in the brain. Endorphin, which was discovered in England in 1975, has exactly the same effect as opium or its refined version, morphine, which is used as an anesthetic. Endorphin reduces physical pain and restores a feeling of well-being. Such phenomena are explained by the fact that this substance attaches itself to the lymbic system of the brain, the center of emotion and instinct, relieving pain and inducing a feeling of intoxication and great happiness.

It has also been suggested that endorphin may have something to do with anesthesia by acupuncture. Experiments have shown that when a needle is inserted into point ST-36 (Figure 1.2) of a monkey's leg, the flow of endorphin in the brain and spinal cord increases. Experiments with rats have shown that the release of endorphin in the brain may also be stimulated by fear. When a rat is dissected immediately after it has been frightened, the endorphin level in the brain is found to have increased. (This may also explain the stories of soldiers feeling no pain when shot in battle.) The secretion of endorphin may also be stimulated by the practice of religious austerities and by vigorous physical exercise. The person practicing religious disciplines (for instance, carrying out a penance that may be physically painful) may experience religious exaltation even while feeling pain. Some Christian sects practice penance in order to subjectively experience the crucifixion of Christ. The devotee, however, experiences a feeling of intoxication and is often unaware of any pain. Even in the penance of walking barefoot on fire, practiced in Japan, the ascetic neither feels the heat nor sustains any burning of the feet. In recent years, a further illustration of the effect of endorphin has been discovered: the intoxication experienced by runners known as jogger's lungs, a result of the regularized and continuous rhythm they develop. The effect, directly attributable to the release of endorphin in the brain, is that the runners feel less fatigue.

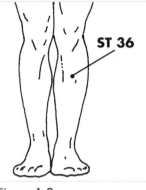

ST 36

Figure 1.2

These examples show that *ki* has profound relevance to the images in a person's mind and that an image has the potential to change the essence and strength of *ki*. When we think about performing a certain task, if we have a positive image of the intended result, the probability of success improves. A positive image increases the flow of *ki* because it heightens its quality. Conversely, fears and anxieties accompanying a negative image decrease the chances of success in the task. The image determines the flow of *ki* and because *ki* influences physical actions and psychological functions, the extent to which a particular image controls our life and well-being is significant.

Kazuyoshi Okada, M.D., reports the following, based on his understanding of life from his own experiences in Zen discipline: "In our daily life we cannot willfully make tears flow, produce saliva and gastric juices, and so on. However, if we use the power of association and imagination, not only can we stimulate the flow of tears and gastric juices, but we can even influence auto-regulating systems such as the heart and blood vessels."[7] This is because our physiological actions are strongly dominated by image. When we imagine a

7. Kazuyoshi Okada, *Seimei no Igaku* [in Japanese] (Osaka: Sogensha, 1989).

frightening situation, our heart beats strongly; when we imagine something terribly sad, tears well up in our eyes. Similarly, people who have experienced eating Japanese pickled plum, the *umeboshi,* merely have to visualize an *umeboshi* and saliva builds up in their mouth. And however hard we try, we cannot willfully stimulate the flow of tears or saliva without conjuring up an image.

Furthermore, the image that people have of themselves is deeply connected to the condition of their health. Significant differences in health and lifestyle are apparent between people who imagine themselves positively and those who imagine themselves negatively. This means that a negative perception of oneself has a negative effect on health. Anxiety and fear suppress the autonomic nervous system and lower the body's resistance to illness. People who harbor negative emotions such as anger and hatred toward others endanger their own health through the acidification of their blood. There is some proof that anger instantly increases blood acid levels. Therefore, all negative images and emotions, toward oneself or others, cause a decrease and stagnation in the flow of *ki* and thereby result in immediate ill health. Therefore, the mind must not be excluded from medical therapy.

As previously mentioned, Simonton therapy uses image suggestion as a main method of cancer treatment. First, the patient is led into a deep state of relaxation. The image suggested is of the white corpuscles accumulating around the cancer cells, consuming them, and carrying them away. It has been reported that when an image is created of the white corpuscles as a large cavalry killing the small, sluggish cancer cells, the malignant tumor stops maturing at a particularly high rate and begins to contract. In this method of therapy, it is extremely important that the patient be completely relaxed. Relaxation heightens the alignment of cells and allows a stronger flow of *ki.* If there is psychological stress, the image and its success are hindered and the results are unsatisfactory. Stress is not caused by imagining a favorable result; it is born from a negative image or premonition of suffering. Therefore optimism is necessary for the success of the image and the cure of illness.

The Interrelationship Between the Mind and Body

There are many different examples of the power of a suggested image. Some people are allergic to the leaves of the lacquer tree (*Rhus verniciflua*). If such a person is covered with leaves from another tree but is told that these leaves are from the lacquer tree, the person will experience a reaction exactly the same as that produced by lacquer leaves. If a person under hypnosis is touched with a cold stick and told that the stick is a red-hot iron, his or her skin will sustain real burns. Similarly, when a person under hypnosis is struck on the back with an ordinary piece of rope and told that it is a snake, impressions of snake scales are left on the skin. Although modern science has witnessed all these experiments and their results, it still does not have the means to understand or accept such phenomena. Yet the relationship between the mind and body is probably more important to the development of medicine of the future than the study of pharmacological effects through tests and experiments on animals.

The mind and body interrelationship cannot be defined solely by prevailing natural laws or scientific experiment. Oriental medicine has long had an understanding of this interrelationship and, in the East, medicine is known as the Art of Benevolence, in which the relationship of faith established with the patient is very much regarded as a significant healing technique. This means that the patient's character and his or her rapport with the healer has profound clinical relevance. It is thought that the effects of even a placebo depend on whether the patient has faith in the doctor who prescribes it. Furthermore, the results may be even more successful if the drug is prescribed by a doctor who also has faith. Each individual has a unique existence, and in the mind-body interrelationship illness too has diverse characteristics. However, science does not consider the individual's inherent characteristics. Rather, it separates the body from the mind and reduces the mind to something that can be quantitatively measured, thereby depriving modern medicine of the consideration of the individual's character. Modern medicine supports the belief in science, which creates a need for the mass production of drugs prescribed for categorized illnesses.

The one branch of modern medicine that has not lost sight of the need to confront people's character is psychoanalysis and psychotherapy. However, because it has attempted to do the impossible—generalizing the human character and expressing it quantitatively—the Western medical world has long been inadequate even in these methods of healing. Western society has had difficulty recognizing the existence of the unconscious. Consequently, psychoanalysis and psychotherapy were ignored by medical science until the end of the last century. In the East, however, great emphasis has traditionally been placed on the unconscious mind in relation to the function of *ki.* Therefore, medical treatment too has been carried out from the point of view of the interrelationship of the mind and body. The reason psychotherapy as we know it did not develop in the East as a separate branch of medicine is that Oriental medicine approaches healing from a holistic point of view whereas psychotherapy focuses only on the mind. In Oriental medicine it is thought that a person with a psychiatric illness has previously suffered some unknown, physical complaint. The treatment, therefore, is based on the patient's subjective symptoms and the belief that treating the body in the very early stages of illness may mean the prevention of serious psychiatric disorders. In contrast, Western medicine does not begin treatment until the illness has been identified and categorized.

Magic, Religion, and Meditation

The word *illness* in Japanese, *byo-ki*, is the ailment of *ki* in the union of the mind and body, and since *ki* is the object of therapy in Oriental medicine, diagnosis is based on the interrelationship of mind and body. In the East, the primary factors that contribute to illness are said to be: anxiety, fear, anger, and other negative emotions, contributing to mental illness; excess work and stress, to physical illness; and environmental pollution and the intake of artificial additives in food, to social illness. The aim of medical treatment is the creation of a better world as a whole through the healing of the individual. Therapy is not meant merely to provide symptomatic relief; it can also help the individual attain his or her karma and purify the world, because the part is equal to the whole. In the therapeutic practices carried out by the ancient shaman, religious rites used for treating illness were not only performed to induce a result based on suggestion, but also used for the ablution of karma.

Even modern, "civilized" people faced with illness expect, deep in their subconscious minds, an element of magic in their medical treatment. This may be due to our subliminal memory of ancient medical therapies. It seems that the altar has merely been replaced by examination machines, the incense by the smell of antiseptic solution, and the spells by the machines with numerous dials used in hospitals.

In France, interesting experiments have been carried out by measuring the brain waves of Buddhist monks during meditation. When monks go into a meditative state, the production of alpha waves is at 8–13 hertz, lower than in normal consciousness. As meditation continues, 4–7 hertz (theta waves) begin to appear. (See Figure 1.3.) It is thought that during meditation, the function of the epithelium is suppressed—therefore activating the midbrain —which increases the conceptualization of contrast and the intuitive perception of life. As a result of meditation, the body's homeostasis is heightened and the cells are tuned into an image of well-being. In Simonton therapy, the patient's relaxed mental condition may be seen as a meditative state. Meditation has been proven to be a significantly effective element of therapy because it is conducive to the use of images to improve the patient's physical health. Obviously, these findings indicate the medical significance of meditation therapy and the need to devote more research time to the significance of spirituality and the mind-body interrelationship in medical treatment.

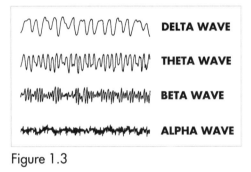

Figure 1.3

The Holistic Approach of Shiatsu Therapy

One aspect of shiatsu therapy is the effect touching the skin has on the midbrain. As mentioned earlier, touching the skin has a direct effect on the lymbic system, which is a part of the midbrain. Through shiatsu therapy, the patient's brain waves change to alpha waves. In the relaxed mental and physical condition induced by appropriate shiatsu therapy, patients release their thoughts and, by the practitioner's hands, can be expected to acquire a positive image of themselves and others.

What is therapeutically significant is that patients are liberated from the negative image previously held. For instance, those who are prone to stomach ailments live with the subconscious image that something is wrong with their stomach, making them constantly aware of their stomach. People with neck stiffness are conscious of their neck region and those with lumbago are conscious of their back region. In other words, one is overly conscious of any one part of the body merely because that particular part of the body has sustained some sort of injury or is for some reason unhealthy. It is an indication that such people have lost contact with the holistic nature of their body. When people are aware of their whole body, they do not create negative images about themselves or their body.

The aim of Oriental training of the body and mind is the personal experience of an indescribable consciousness that merges with the universe and the realization that the self exists as one with nature. The purpose of shiatsu therapy is the restoration of the holistic nature of the patient's body and mind and a condition where peace and harmony replace physical and mental health disorders. Patients are liberated from negative self-images and are able to begin true self-realization through their own world experiences. In other words, an important aspect of shiatsu therapy is leading patients on the road to self-realization.

Compassion

It is thought that the best way of relieving stress is to feel appreciation and compassion toward others. The patient who is appreciative of therapy—shiatsu or even hospital medicine—heals more quickly. Appreciation restrains the patient's pessimistic feelings about the illness, which in turn puts patients at ease, pulls their cells into alignment, and enables their body to draw in more universal *ki* energy. When we receive universal *ki* with positive feelings, such as compassion, the circulation of positive, healthy energy is generated. On the other hand, when we receive universal energy with negative feelings, do not offer appreciation and compassion to others, and use the energy for self-love, *ki* stagnates, fears and anxieties are born, and the mind and body are in a state of tension.

The World Health Organization (WHO) proposes that "being healthy means being mentally, physically, and socially healthy." The road to mental, physical, and social health and well-being is opened when there is positive and constructive direction of universal *ki* toward everyone and everything. The WHO definition of health is also appropriate as a definition of "welfare" or "happiness." Medical philosophy is something that should not only contribute to the welfare of humanity, but also direct each individual on the road to good health and happiness. The essence of Oriental medicine is the quest for harmony with nature and the significance of true health is the discovery of harmony with everyone and everything. From this point of view, happiness, welfare, and good health are one and the same thing. When one is lost, we realize its importance for the first time and become restless and unsettled.

In ancient China, a doctor was considered a person who healed the entire community or country. Medicine need not only exist for the cure and treatment of a person's body as though repairing a machine. Medicine should use the opportunity of treating illness to direct the individual toward the most appropriate way of life, contributing to the self-realization of the individual. It is at this point that medicine is linked to religion. This does not mean that medicine should become involved with any one particular religion or set of beliefs. It does, however, need to contribute to people's happiness and self-realization, and it needs to value such emotions as love and compassion for the health of humanity, which ultimately means the health of the planet.

Doin-Ankyo and the Art of Immortality

The Significance of Different Therapies

Shiatsu originated in *doin-ankyo*, which held a central place among the various methods of medical treatment, such as acupuncture and infusions, used in ancient China. *Doin* includes meditation techniques such as *qigong*, which emphasizes physical exercise through the effort of the individual. *Ankyo* is a therapeutic technique using correction and pressure that depends on the efforts of another person, namely the practitioner. The practice of *doin* and *ankyo* emerged from the prevailing environmental conditions in which all living things in China (the center of the world, according to Chinese philosophy) were born. The Classics of Oriental medicine note that the preferred methods of therapy differed according to the environment in which people lived. For instance, in the extremely cold northern regions, moxibustion was the principal means of therapy. On the other hand, medical therapies that made use of needles developed in the warmer southern regions. Likewise, medicinal plants were used in treatment in the western areas because of the high consumption of meat and dairy products, while bloodletting and the use of lithic needles developed on the eastern coastal regions, where the principal diet was fish with a high intake of salt.

There are two reasons why *doin-ankyo* was recognized as the basis of medical treatment in ancient China. One is that these practices led to the discovery of the concept of meridians, which was later to become the basis of Chinese medicine. The second reason underlies the fundamental concept of Chinese medicine: to follow nature faithfully. *Doin-ankyo* is a gentle, natural technique carried out by the application of people's hands, which, as in acupuncture and moxibustion, does not injure the living body and does not intrude in or obstruct its natural functions. Because Oriental medicine perceives the cause of illness as a blockage in the circulation of energy along the meridians, the aim of medical treatment is to facilitate this circulation. Even in cases where there is an obvious external cause for disease, it is believed that unless there is a disturbance in the vital force, the disease will not invade the internal part of the body.[8] Therefore, more than simply treating symptoms, the Rules of Health of *ankyo* and *doin* emphasize healing from the very source of life.

The Classics state: "*Ki* is upset and uprises in times of anger, and vanishes in moments of sadness. *Ki* is excessively low when one is frightened, and when one thinks too much, *ki* has no outlet and becomes blocked." In other words, stagnation in the flow of *ki* is not only caused by stress and fatigue but also by oppressive, negative emotions and prejudices. Such emotions generate disorders in *ki,* causing disturbances in normal meridianal circulation. When *ki* stagnates, there is an imbalance of the living body within nature, hindering response to changes in the natural environment.

According to the Classics, the origin of all illness is the inability of the living body to respond to natural environmental changes. The practices of *doin-ankyo* restore meridianal circulation, heal disorders in the living body, and foster a harmonious state of exchange between *ki* and nature. Those who practice these disciplines are liberated from negative emotions and spiritual oppression and are led to the awakening of their inner nature. As a result, they are able to maintain flexibility in mind and body and respond to any

---

8. *Naisho nakereba gaijanashi* is a Japanese proverb that means "where there is no internal scar, there is no external evil."

changes in the environment. In the Eastern tradition, true freedom was said to come from understanding and attaining this flexibility. Those who have awakened to this freedom as a human ideal are recognized as sages.

A sage is not simply someone with a noble mind or advanced soul. A sage is someone who listens to and obediently follows his inner nature. The Chinese character for sage is made up of two characters meaning "ear" and "to develop." A sage listens with the heart to his inner voice without letting the ego interfere. There is a proverb relating to Oriental diagnosis, "the sage is one who knows by listening." Here, sage refers to the selfless mind that captures and becomes filled with the essence of nature. It suggests a clear mental state in which the healer can actually feel the patient's personal concerns and the invisible disturbances in *ki* that underlie the symptoms. The sage's mind is one that does not discriminate between the self and others. Originally, the union with Tao was the objective of Oriental philosophy and medicine. Throughout *The Yellow Emperor's Classic of Internal Medicine,* the union with Tao is held as the ideal of human character and is always used to describe the sage, who exists as one with Tao where the union of internal and external nature can be witnessed.

Doin-Ankyo and Shiatsu

As mentioned previously, *doin* is a general term for the technique of releasing meridianal flow through one's own efforts. Also included in the term *doin* are *qigong* (which has recently gained popularity in China) and *tai-chi.* According to one scholar of *sendo, qigong* was a part of the *sendo* discipline and was introduced after gaining the support of modern medicine. Like *sendo,* the ultimate purpose of *qigong* is the ability to control the freedom of meridianal circulation in the macrocosmic circuit throughout the body. *Ankyo,* which releases meridianal flow through the manual massage technique, is a word that came about from combining the words *anma* (massage) and *kyosei* (manipulation). Therefore *anma,* the predecessor of shiatsu, includes the posture-correction techniques of chiropractic and osteopathy. However, as Shizuto Masunaga points out, the massage techniques carried out in ancient China were not vastly different from the gentle pounding technique of modern massage. In order to actually feel the meridians, the healer must be in sympathy with the patient and, rather than using the soft pounding, must maintain a constant steady pressure with the hands (chapter 2). This has become the fundamental technique of shiatsu therapy.[9]

Scholars previously thought that shiatsu was merely a means of awakening the patient's vitality. However, with increased research, we have come to understand that this is very similar to *doin*—a means of enriching the life force of the healer. By systematizing this as the "principle of *ki* shiatsu," shiatsu therapy became a discipline with the purpose of integrating heightened universal *ki* with the practitioner's own life force. As a result, scholars have come to understand why *ankyo* and *doin* were treated as one rather than separately in ancient China. *Ankyo*, as shiatsu performed for the sake of the other (patient), becomes *doin* to oneself (healer). The type of shiatsu called *Tao shiatsu*, which is said to awaken the unitary force of all living things, arose from the method of healing that incorporates the principles of *doin-ankyo*.

The Art of Immortality

In the existing classical records, *doin-ankyo* is categorized as the Art of Immortality. *Sendo* too was originally known as the Art of Immortality. *Sendo* and *doin-ankyo* have been developed as methods of medical health care that promote perennial youth and longevity. In Oriental medicine, the idea of medically treating a person after the onset of illness is considered similar to manufacturing weapons after a war has commenced. This surprising comparison is indicative of the serious emphasis placed on the prevention of mental and physical illness rather than on the treatment of existing illness. Passive prevention, however, is not enough. The goal of health care is universal vitality: the prevention of aging, freeing the mind from negativity, and the attainment of spiritual enlightenment. The Classics note that the Art of Immortality perfects the vital force, erases spiritual vexation, surpasses the obstacles of life and death, and relieves pressures and restraints. Health care therefore includes not only prevention and cure of illness but also spiritual self-discipline. In Western medicine, where physical disease is cured by drugs and prevented through public health and mental disorder is dealt with through counseling, the individual cannot find a therapeutic balance be-

---

9. Shizuto Masunaga, *Zen Shiatsu* (Tokyo: Japan Publications, 1977). This is an English edition of *Shiatsu*, which was published in Japanese by Idon Nihonsha in 1974.

tween the spiritual, the mental, and the physical. Oriental medicine does not treat individual problems separately as does Western medicine; rather, it treats everything holistically and harmoniously.

In the Classics, the Art of Immortality is expressed as follows: "Preserve the truth or purity (*shin*) of life and search for freedom (*yu*)." "The truth of life" refers to the union of the mind and body. Through the understanding of this union, a person becomes one with universal *ki*, which enriches his or her life force. When there is a union of mind and body, disturbance and exhaustion of *ki* are avoided. Since ancient times in Japan the sayings "disciplining the abdomen" and "being able to discipline the *tanden*" have been used to mean that the union of the mind and body can be attained by replenishing the energy in the *tanden* area of the lower abdomen. *Yu* means to have the potential to open one's mind and to fuse with nature. In everyday life, the role of *yu* is the return to a creative freedom and flexibility away from the thought and action patterns of work. The result of the union with universal life is that the body and mind must reach a state of *yu*, and that in this state of freedom and flexibility, the mind and body are able to respond to any changes.

In ancient China, the Art of Immortality was said to be a method of attaining eternal youth. Physically, this meant longevity and youth of the body. Psychologically, it signified an awakening to eternal life as a means of understanding spiritual immortality. The awakening to eternal life is the intuitive understanding of the mutually contradictory phenomena of life (yin) and death (yang) and their shared origin. This is an awakening to Tao, the fundamental aim of the various martial arts and religions of the East.

Non-Action in Nature

Sages are able to preserve the purity of life because they are usually in a state of *yu*. Their every act conforms to the Tao—Way of the Universe (in Buddhist terms, *Dharma*). Lao-Tzu called this "non-action in nature."[10] This is the liberation of the self from the selfish motives of all actions. Unlike the prevailing ideologies of Western cultures, "non-action in nature" de-emphasizes the individual and excludes focus on the ego. Since Oriental medicine sees the

---

10. Non-action in nature, *mu-i-shi-zen*. The character *mu* (*wu* in Chinese) means void or nothingness. The "spirit of nothingness" is fundamental to Chinese philosophy and Buddhist doctrines.

original cause of illness as existing in the patient's self (in other words as something created by the ego), it aims to remove the ego in order to discover the patient's inner natural strength. Treatment in Oriental medicine takes place through the conceptualization and personal experience of "non-action in nature" from the point of view of both the patient and the healer. The Classics state that the practice of *doin-ankyo* is particularly effective in liberating egoistic prejudices and awakening the patient to the immortality of life.

Teate: Touch Therapy

The Significance of Touch

The *manual technique* of medical therapy literally means curing illness through touch, without the use of implements or drugs. Manual therapy exists throughout the world and is by no means limited to shiatsu. Since ancient times, sages and many other shamanistic and spiritual healers have cured illness simply by touching the patient's body. However, the act of touching the affected area of the body is not limited specifically to religious practice; we all unconsciously touch areas of pain in our body. If we have an acute external injury, chronic illness, or pain, we instinctively touch the area with our hands. The first explanation for this behavior that comes to mind is that we are instinctively trying to stop the bleeding and perhaps, by touching the source of chronic pain or stiffness with our hand, promote the circulation of blood in the area, which may improve the condition. Shizuto Masunaga claims that the manual technique of therapy began with the substitution of a healer's hand for one's own.

What is the psychological significance of touching an ailing part of the body with one's own hands? When young children, who have as yet undeveloped egos and cannot differentiate between the self and others, fall down and hurt themselves, they do not touch the painful area with their hands, but merely cry and want to snuggle against their mother's bosom. It could perhaps be said that the comfort of mother's arms is more important than the instinctive action of touching the affected area. Children run to their mother's arms because of a condition of inseparability that exists between mother and child; we all instinctively want to return to the womb where, we subconsciously remember, we never experienced any pain or anxiety. The instinct of wanting to snuggle against the mother's bosom may be the desire to return to a state where there is total freedom from pain, fear, and ego. This may be the manifestation of the wish to return to nature, similar to the instinct for touching with the hands (*teate*). Lao-Tzu too preached that "people's well-being depends on their ability to return to nature," and the *teate* technique of healing signifies the restoration of health through the personal experience of the union with nature of both the patient and the healer.

Doctors, Shamans, and Spiritual Healers

In modern Japanese, the word *teate* has become a synonym for medical healing practices because all medical therapy is specifically based on the manual technique. While touching the patient's body, healers throughout the ages have prayed for and summoned the spiritual powers of the gods, thereby healing those burdened with pain and suffering. It is for this reason that the healer was once recognized as the shaman or medium and known to have spiritual healing powers. Illness has long been cured by the mysterious powers of the shamans. The fact that medical healing initially took place side by side with religious rites shows that it was understood to be beyond the patient's physiology. In the West, during the Middle Ages, monasteries were established as places of medical research, and science and religion were inextricably linked. Perhaps patients expect their healers to be potential mediums because they are in awe of anyone who understands the extraordinary cause or origin of an illness, something the patient knows nothing about. In other words, when we come in contact with the extraordinary world, psychologically we are able to recognize the mysterious spiritual world. The spiritual medium or shaman intervenes between the ordinary world (the world of people) and the extraordinary world (that of spirits) and imparts the oracle in a state of trance (possessed by spirits) in order to cure illness. It is through this process that healing initially took place.

Spiritual healing was the original form of medical therapy. The English word *medicine*, which signifies drugs and medical science, derives from the word *medium*. (The word *meditation* also originates from *medium*.) The medium was a magician who burned incense and chanted incantations. He wore masks and feathers, often dressed as a woman, and danced, possessed by spirits. Then, following the various religious rites, he prayed to the spirits or the gods and cured patients with his spiritual powers. The medium led people into the spiritual world and played the role of mediator between the ordinary world of people and the extraordinary world of the gods.

According to Taro Nakayama, the original word for medicine was symbolized by the Chinese character shown in Figure 1.4, which has been simplified to 医. 匚 represents the bed on which the sick person lies. 矢 is the arrow that shoots the evil spirit carrying the illness. 殳 represents the altar and 巫 is the shaman or medium. The upper horizontal line of 巫 represents heaven and the lower line, earth. The medium (巫者, *fu-sha*) is the link between both heaven and earth. The fact that there are two characters for person, 人, indicates that with the union of the medium and the patient, a spiritual exchange between heaven and earth takes place.[11]

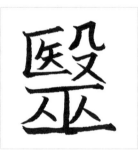

Figure 1.4

The Art of Benevolence

In Oriental medicine, the concept of the Art of Benevolence, which has been handed down for millennia, expresses the spirit of medical therapy based on the union of the healer and the patient.[12] It is said that medical therapy should take place through dialogue between the souls of two living people. Patients make a lengthy report of their symptoms so that the healer may understand the personality that has fallen into the extraordinary world known as pain, a world of social isolation and helplessness. Patients need their heal-

---

11. Taro Nakayama, *Nihon Mikoshi* [in Japanese] (Tokyo: Dai Okayama Shoten, 1980).
12. The character for benevolence (*jin*) represents the union between two people.

er to acknowledge their suffering and sympathize with them so that they may be liberated from their psychological isolation. Medical therapy has the capacity to incorporate the Art of Benevolence, through which the patient can return from the extraordinary world of pain to a healthy normality.

The spirit of the Art of Benevolence is absent in modern medicine, which insists on treating the patient objectively. If people have begun to turn their back on modern medical science, it is because it focuses solely on the physical aspect of the body, neglecting a person's spirituality. This spiritual neglect not only means a lack of consideration for the psychological origin of illness but also reflects a lack of psychological support for the patient's return from suffering.

Even in modern, highly developed civilizations, people who become ill look subconsciously for the image of the ancient shaman in the doctor, exemplifying that every illness is haunted by the shadow of death and that the focus of medical therapy should be the healing of the soul. Because modern medicine developed through a focus on emergency treatment, such as in war, it tends to put too little emphasis on spiritual healing. However, in every occurrence of illness, patients consciously or subconsciously hope that their body and mind will be treated as one and that their suffering will be sympathized with and their soul liberated.

Teate: **The Medical Therapy of Touch**

The action of touching the patient's body is the expression of the mind of the healer who prays for the cure of the illness. It has been reported from actual experiments conducted throughout the world that when healers perform manual therapy, a certain amount of energy is released from their hands. For example, the Kirlian photographs stand as proof for the existence of the aura. S. D. and V. K. Kirlian discovered that one type of energy emitted by the human body takes the form of ultraviolet rays. They took high voltage photos of the electrical discharge or *corona* emitted from the skin and reported that there was a difference in the photographs of a spiritual healer before and after the practice of healing was conducted.

Furthermore, Kanjitsu Iijima claims that over one hundred years ago the German anatomist Franz Anton Mesmer had already detected radiation emanating from the palm of the hand. He reported that an enzyme that was like a tiny gun discharging fifty thousand bullets in each finger was responsible for this radiation. He also reported that this discharge differs according to the individuals and their emotional state, said to be discharged more readily in someone with a "loving heart."[13] The force that radiates from the palm of the hand to heal illness has long been used throughout the world. It has also been reported that the suffering of patients in the final stages of cancer can be relieved by the simple touch of a hand. Many people were miraculously healed by Christ in the Bible by hearing his words, receiving his touch, or touching his robe. It is thought that these phenomena are due to the *ki* released by the great teacher, who was filled with the universal energy of love.

In *qigong* therapy, practiced in China, the *ki* accumulated in the healer's *tanden* radiates from the palm of the hand to cure illness. However, in shiatsu, the therapy is such that patients accumulate *ki* in their own *tanden*, in conformity with the *ki* that radiates from the healer's hand and in simultaneous exchange with the *ki* of heaven. *Ki* is called *prana* in India. It is said that strong *prana* generated by the concentration of a particular thought during prayer can cause changes in the arrangement of atoms and the energy field of physical structures.

People who have a strong exchange with the *ki* of the universe also breathe deeply, are in a relaxed state, have an increased metabolism, and are healthy. In Zen, yoga, and *sendo*, the purpose of the training in breathing methods is to enhance the exchange with the *ki* of the universe, which is facilitated through controlled breathing. Those who practice these disciplines are also spiritually at peace and are able to give love freely to others. On the other hand, those who have a weak exchange with the *ki* of the universe are lost in gloom, filled with unrest, and focused on self-love. In our daily life we encounter many different people and, depending on the type of person we are, we project positive or negative feelings to those around us. If a healthy tree is planted beside a withered tree, the withered tree will return to good health. It could be said that *ki* has a similar mutual interaction.

Individuality is the point of difference in the reflection of the energy of the universe. We all maintain our vitality by receiving *ki* from its universal source. However, we each create a difference in the *ki* we generate through our own self-image and the image we have of the outside world. Human existence may be explained as a mirror that reflects each person's universal *ki*. If the mirror is foggy or dirty, it cannot reflect light; a negative image distorts

13. Iijima Kanjitsu, *Bukkyo Yoga Nyumon* [in Japanese] (Tokyo: Nichibo Shuppansha, 1973).

the reflection of universal energy. When a person's soul is purified and the original *ki* of the universe is reflected as positive energy, deep love energy flows from that person. Depending on their strength, such people may have an effect on everyone, from people in their immediate vicinity to people all around the world.

The liberation of the purified spirit and a strong positive *ki* have the power to cure illness. Therefore, like Christ, the sage who is in a state of union with the love of the universe has the capacity to instantly initiate an exchange of *ki* with the sick people simply by allowing them to touch his robe, at which time the sick people are purged and filled with life force and their ailment is cured. *Teate*, the original form of medical treatment, is dependent on this type of exchange of *ki*. In other words, the exchange of *ki* with the universe through the healer's hands fills the patient with life and returns the patient to a state of physical, mental, and spiritual balance and well-being.

Chapter Two

Basic Techniques

The Various Techniques of Shiatsu

Definition of Shiatsu

Shiatsu may be defined as a method of therapy that cures illness and promotes good health through the patient's exchange of *ki* with nature, which takes place through a medium (the healer) who is in sympathy with the patient's response to the applied pressure. The word *shiatsu* came into use in Japan during the Taisho period (1912–1926). Its meaning is easily understood from the characters used: *shi* means finger and *atsu* means pressure. In Japan, after the war, the various folk remedies that had until then been in use were legislated and all manual therapeutic techniques except *anma* and massage were designated as "shiatsu."

There are some who think that because of its name (finger pressure), shiatsu traditionally involves only the application of pressure by the fingers, and in particular the thumbs. However, shiatsu is a method that, through the application of pressure, promotes sympathy between patient and healer. Furthermore, the knees and elbows, which are naturally included in the shiatsu technique, may be used as well as the fingers, as long as they are used effectively. It was from this perspective that Masunaga developed the formal shiatsu techniques.

Shiatsu Techniques

1. **Palm Pressure.** The whole palm of the hand is used on the face, back, abdomen, and legs. The healer uses palm pressure to recognize and understand the condition of the patient's entire body through the whole palm of the hand. With palm pressure, it is possible to give soft pressure to a wide area.

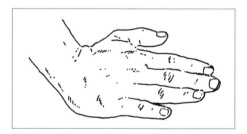

1. Palm pressure

2. **Heel of the Hand Pressure.** The healer focuses his or her *ki* on the heel of the hand. This method is used on the head and legs, where it is possible to apply strong, stable pressure.

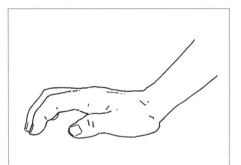

2. Heel of the hand pressure

3. **Grasping Pressure (*ha-aku-atsu*).** The character *ha* represents the shape of a snake zigzagging across the ground. *Aku* means to close tightly. Therefore, grasping pressure is applied by adhering tightly to the patient's body with the whole palm of the hand. Grasping pressure is not applied by simply concentrating on one part of the patient's body but by visualizing the *ki* in the patient's whole body. This method is used on areas such as the neck.

4. **Thumb Pressure.** This is the most popular of all shiatsu techniques. Although it is known as thumb pressure, it must be performed in collaboration with the other four fingers. Thumb pressure alone triggers stress in the sympathetic nerves, which is the opposite of the desired result. This method is used on the back and in meridianal therapy.

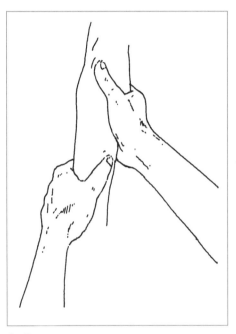

3. Grasping pressure

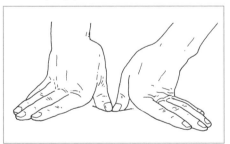

4. Thumb pressure

5. **Index Finger Pressure.** The healer places the middle finger on the index finger and applies pressure using both fingers together. This is used to determine the *tsubo*.

6. **Four Finger Pressure.** The healer places the middle finger on the *tsubo* and applies pressure with the force of all four fingers. This method is used in meridianal therapy and *hara* diagnosis (chapter 4).

7. **Elbow Pressure.** There are two types of elbow pressure: one uses the elbow and the other uses the ulna (called ulna pressure). In the latter, the pressure is applied gently. This method is used on the back and in meridianal therapy.

8. **Knee Pressure.** Although this is called knee pressure, it is the part of the leg below the knee, not the head of the knee, that is used. The healer supports his or her own weight on both hands. When this method is practiced correctly, it is possible to give a pleasant feeling of pressure over a wide area. This method is used on both the arms and the legs.

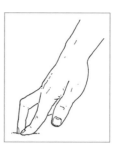

5. Index finger pressure

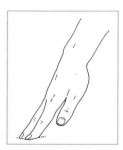

6. Four finger pressure

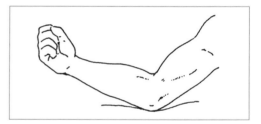

7. Elbow pressure

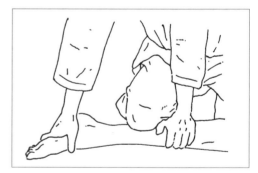

8. Knee pressure

9. **Middle Finger Tip Pressure.**
The healer places the index finger on the middle finger and
applies pressure using these
two fingers together. This
method is used in *tsubo* therapy
on the neck, the side of the face,
and other parts of the head.

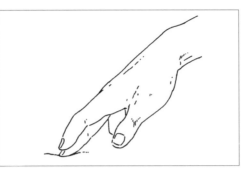

9. Middle finger tip pressure

10. **Second Knuckle of the Middle
Finger Pressure.** This knuckle is
used for continuous pressure
on the *tsubo.*

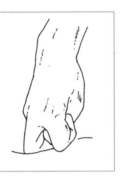

10. Second knuckle of
the middle finger
pressure

11. **Second Knuckle of the Index
Finger Pressure.** The thumb
and second knuckle of the
index finger are used simultaneously. This method is used in
shiatsu on children.

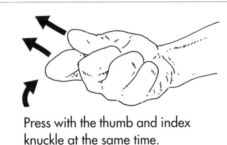

Press with the thumb and index
knuckle at the same time.

11. Second knuckle of the index finger
pressure

Projection and Support Methods of Applying Pressure

Regardless of which technique is used, the characteristics of shiatsu therapy always include both the *projection technique* (*sha*) of applying pressure and the
support technique (*ho*) to sustain it. In therapy, the projection hand applies pressure, but what is of utmost importance is the function of the support hand. The

support hand does the work of yin, maintaining the whole body, and the projection hand does the work of yang, functioning on the surface. Novices often mistakenly direct their consciousness only to the moving function of the projection technique, neglecting the importance of support. This is probably because the projection technique functions consciously, while the support technique is unconscious. The secrets of Eastern martial arts lie in the unification of yin and yang and the unification of the conscious and the unconscious. In shiatsu therapy too, the techniques of support and projection are a union carried out by the integration of *ki*, which unifies the conscious and the unconscious.

To practice this type of shiatsu, one must first learn the basic forms of whole-body shiatsu. The Oriental disciplines of martial arts and healing arts begin with understanding form. It is in the fusion of form that the spirit and techniques of the Old Masters are concentrated. Through learning and repeating the form and knowledge of basic whole-body shiatsu, it is not only possible to attain spiritual and technical standards equal to those of the Old Masters but also possible to practice all the techniques unconsciously. This is the ultimate introduction to the world of *ki*. What Lao-Tzu called "non-action in nature" is the disappearance of all artificiality from a person's conduct. Shiatsu, too, is considered a type of "non-active" function in nature because its true basic techniques can be practiced unconsciously once its form has been studied and adopted.

The importance of learning and using form precisely can be seen in the movements of *tai-chi*, where form establishes one current throughout the body. Some students and practitioners have changed the basic form of shiatsu suit their own ideas, but the unexceptional creativity of such people stops midway. This is because each aspect of form is like an individual stone in a wall: if one stone slides out of place the whole wall will collapse. Form is not something that can be put together or modified piece by piece. It exists as a current and as a whole. This is not to say that each aspect does not have its specific therapeutic significance. The basic technique of whole-body shiatsu is not a practice that is fixed in form. Rather, the study of shiatsu based on the principles of *ki* and the understanding of the mind actually surpasses form. Zen, which also begins with the study of form, preaches that once the mind understands form, the individual enters a world that surpasses it.

As mentioned previously, understanding Eastern martial arts, which also include the art of healing, begins with acquiring knowledge of a spiritual phase that brings form into existence through repetitive training. Once one acquires the mind of Tao, if one is content with the point of view that freely manipulates the traditional form as it is, a form that surpasses tradition is also born. In Zen and *Bushido* this is called "transcendence," and it is a new form that is added to the tradition. Tao is infinite; therefore, the possibility of artistic development and the creation of new forms emerges when one attains the mind of Tao. However, this can only take place when one has reached a level equal to, or surpassing, that of the Old Masters.

Kyo-Jitsu/Ho-Sha

Kyo-jitsu/ho-sha is the most fundamental ideology of Oriental medicine. *Kyo* is a condition in which the patient exhibits a deficiency in vital energy. *Jitsu* is the reverse condition, in which there is an excess of vital energy (chapters 3 and 4). In Oriental medicine, illness is said to be the result when vital energy tends toward one or the other of these two extremes. Therefore, in diagnosis, the healer must first ascertain whether the condition is *kyo* or *jitsu*. A patient with insufficient energy is called *kyosho* (in other words, the yin-type patient) and one with excess energy is called *jissho* (the yang-type patient).

A *kyosho* patient is said to have become ill because of a weakened ability to adjust to the outside world. Healing takes place when health is restored by the *ho* (support) method, which aims to supplement the insufficient energy. The *jissho* patient, whose *ki* has generally stagnated because of excess energy, is treated with the stimulating *sha* (projection) method. This restores balance by projecting the excess energy elsewhere, thereby leading *jissho* patients into relaxation where healing can take place. *Jissho* may be explained as a condition similar to a road so congested with cars that no one can move. *Kyosho* is like a road that has deteriorated to the extent that cars have difficulty traveling along it.

The *jitsu* pattern is most prevalent in sturdy, muscular people, whereas the *kyo* pattern can usually be found among patients with a weak constitution. However, caution must be taken in diagnosis, because there are yang-*kyosho* patients who at first glance appear to be *jissho* and yin-*jissho* patients who appear to be *kyosho*. The *jissho* patient is a reminder that even people with excess energy may become ill, due to their inability to release the excess energy and relax. When energy cannot flow freely, it interferes with the functions of the mind and body. Insufficient exercise is detrimental because energy taken in as food is not consumed and becomes a burden to the body. The Classics state that the patient who is filled with toxins is *jitsu*. Therapy transfers the toxins elsewhere by the *sha* method, and the *ki* that has stagnated due to excess energy is allowed to flow freely once more.

In therapy, it is essential to remember that *jissho* patients have the strength to repel even strong, therapeutic stimulation. Techniques such as acupuncture and moxibustion, which cause some damage to the body, are *sha* methods and appropriate for the *jissho* patient because they involve the use of physical force and strong stimulation. *Jissho* patients are characteristically active and even when their symptoms are severe, they recover quickly. *Kyosho* patients, on the other hand, easily contract chronic illness and take much longer to heal; therefore, cautious consideration must be taken in therapy. *Kyosho* patients have low resistance to stimulation, and strong stimulating therapy may upset their physical balance. When a patient claims to have been unable to stand up the day after receiving treatment, it is because the patient is *kyosho* and the treatment was strong, stimulating *sha* therapy.

If pain from the shiatsu persists until the day after therapy, except in particular circumstances, the therapy must be considered incorrect. Evidence of excess or deficiencies in the patient's whole body and the degree of stimulation of *ho* and *sha* techniques must always be adjusted according to the patient's response to pressure. The skillful shiatsu practitioner is able to read the patient's response to each application of pressure and offer the patient the most appropriate amount of pressure.

Integration of *Ho-Sha* in Shiatsu

The *ho* method of pressure is carried out by the hand that supports the patient's body and the *sha* method by the hand (or knee or elbow) that provides the pressure (Figure 2.12). Every application of pressure in shiatsu involves both the *ho* and *sha* techniques. (When applying pressure with the thumbs, the four fingers do the work of *ho*, and the thumbs do that of *sha*.) The integration of the *ho* and *sha* techniques means that the *ho* and *sha* hands always provide exactly the same degree of pressure. Therefore, when applying constant steady pressure, for instance, both hands must always be felt as one, meaning that the patient is not aware of space between the healer's two hands applying the pressure. In normal states of consciousness, because the discriminatory senses perceive distinctions clearly, the touch of the hands is not felt as one. However, the integration of the *ho-sha* techniques dulls the discriminatory senses and enhances a state of consciousness where there is no feeling of separateness between the subject and object. At such times, not only are the *ho* and *sha* hands felt as one but it is also possible for the healer and the patient to unite and eliminate the distinction between themselves.

In terms of yin and yang, the supporting *ho* hand is yin, and the *sha* hand, which has the active function of applying pressure, is yang. Because yin signifies the whole body, *ho* is more than simply the technique that supports *sha*; it also supports the healer's body and can be better described as the channel through which the healer perceives the patient's response to pressure. When applying pressure through the integration of the *ho-sha* technique, the healer's body is united with the patient's body and shiatsu is performed not as the conscious act of applying pressure by physical strength but as the unconscious act of healing by using *ki*. Through this it is possible to provide the type of shiatsu that generates changes in the patient's body with each application of pressure. The actual experience of the integration of *ho-sha* is equivalent to that of the integration of yin and yang proposed in

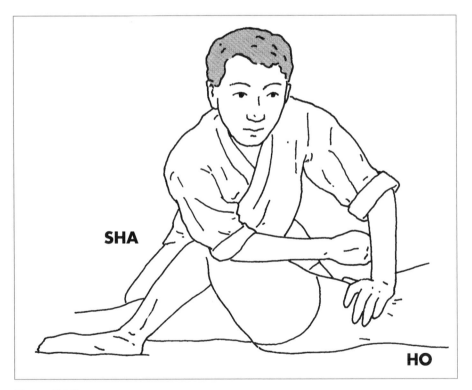

Figure 2.12

Eastern philosophy. It is the sensation of the world of *ki* at the source of existence, which surpasses all antagonism and contradiction.

The Three Principles of Shiatsu

Shiatsu therapy has been developed from the manual techniques of the ancient shamans as a therapeutic method using pressure. According to the appropriate stimulating pressure, "touching the skin" in shiatsu affects the patient both psychologically and physiologically. In Masunaga's detailed explanation of the degree and type of physiological effects induced by shiatsu, he claims that the continuous steady pressure of shiatsu facilitates blood circulation and stimulates metabolism and the flow of body fluids.[1] Shiatsu promotes the function of internal organs by guiding the patient into a condition of heightened responsiveness. Such a condition is important because the patient's responses are generally suppressed due to tension in the sympathetic nerves, which also hinders the function of the internal organs. Therefore, one aim of shiatsu is to liberate the whole body from the stress in the sympathetic nerves. This promotes relaxation, activates the functions of the internal organs, and increases metabolism, allowing the patient a speedy recovery from illness.

There are misconceptions about shiatsu therapy. Some people are led to believe that an illness can be cured simply by pressing a particular *tsubo*, unaware that *tsubo* do not exist in any fixed position. Some also believe that applying pressure to a certain area of the body will cure a particular illness because certain *tsubo* affect certain illnesses. Naturally the results are not effective. Healing through shiatsu does not simply mean applying the appropriate pressure; the healer must also locate the correct *tsubo* with a sympathetic mind toward the patient's vital forces. Masunaga proposes that there are three principles of correct pressure application in the shiatsu method. These principles, which are explained below, are: sustained pressure, continuous steady pressure, and perpendicular pressure.[2]

---

1.   Shizuto Masunaga, *Shiatsu Ryoho* [in Japanese] (Osaka: Sogensha, 1960).
2.   Ibid.

Sustained Pressure

There are those who think that shiatsu uses the pressure of strength accumulated in the thumbs. However, when the shiatsu healer presses onto the patient's body entirely with his or her own strength, the patient's body becomes defensive, creating a condition of stress in the sympathetic nerves. The initial aim of shiatsu is to lead the patient into a condition of heightened responsiveness. Therefore the first principle of shiatsu is sustained pressure, in which the healer does not use muscular strength but supports his or her hand and leans toward the patient as though to use his or her whole body weight (Figure 2.13). One aim of sustained pressure is the opening up of the patient's mind to receive the healer's pressure. The stress is released from the body and the *tsubo* become susceptible to the healer's pressure. This allows the effects of the pressure to reach the depths of the patient's mind, thereby inducing a state of relaxation.

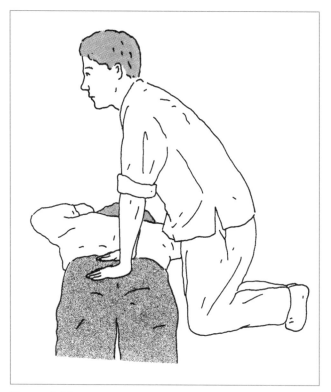

Figure 2.13

The art of relaxation, in therapy as well as daily human interactions, is by no means unique to shiatsu. Patients are able to relax by responding to the healer's relaxed state and healers who want their patients to relax must first of all be relaxed themselves. Being in a relaxed state means being in a defenseless condition and breathing deeply and fully. This is a state in which the self is opened to nature; shiatsu therapy can only be performed in such a state. Our skin is the boundary between ourselves and others. When someone seems to want to harm our body, the body immediately tries to defend itself: the sympathetic nerves harden and go into a state of tension. This is why probing and overzealous pressure are not appropriate in shiatsu.

Because the relaxation of the patient is the primary consideration in shiatsu therapy, it is essential that the healer is first of all relaxed and receptive to nature. Anyone can feel at ease in the presence of a defenseless being. For instance, one's blood pressure may drop when one sits beside a pet simply because one is influenced by the relaxed, defenseless state of the animal. A child is also a defenseless being. When a child leans toward us, we respond by offering support. In the sustained pressure technique, the healer leans on the patient's body in the same way as the defenseless child leans on the adult. What Masunaga calls sustained pressure is the patient's response of trying to support the healer. The defenseless feeling of leaning toward another is the manifestation of utmost and complete faith in the other; the patient surrenders his or her own body to the responsibility of the healer.

Having faith and becoming passive toward another is the fundamental therapeutic ideology of Oriental medicine. Furthermore, the healer's faith in the patient is characteristic of therapies that make the patient the subject rather than the object. Patients' faith functions internally, signifying the faith they have in their own power of healing, that is, in their own vital force. Also, because patients ultimately draw on their own inherent healing powers, healers must not attempt to reform their patients or treat them aggressively. In other words, the healer adopts a relatively passive role and becomes sympathetic toward the patient's life energies. Shiatsu, acupuncture, and Chinese herbal medicine, the original forms of Oriental medicine, are mediating techniques through which the healer sympathizes with the patient's life.

The main aim of Western medicine is to relieve symptoms, by administering drugs and performing surgery. These healing methods correct patients by so-called medical cures and place them in a position of complete submission. Unlike Oriental medicine, which considers the significance of the

symptoms to the body, Western medicine observes the symptoms and immediately tries to relieve them aggressively. Therefore the doctor is never
passive toward the patient as in Oriental medicine. In Western medicine,
symptoms must have abnormal numerical readings that can be discovered
through analysis; otherwise, they cannot be categorized and are therefore
not recognized. Such uncategorizable subjective symptoms are disregarded
and attributed to the imagination, and drugs for psychological instability are
prescribed.

In Oriental medicine, and particularly Tao shiatsu, therapy is limited entirely to the patient's subjective symptoms. In cases where the patient does
not have subjective symptoms, if a meridianal disorder is recognized, it is
identified as a symptom, and it is possible to cure such a disorder before it is
manifested as illness. Oriental medicine has long claimed that "the sage
cures before illness takes place." The most effective medical treatment that
practices this type of healing is meridianal shiatsu. Everyone has potential
meridianal disorders indicated by changes in the individual's vitality from
the shifting balance of yin and yang. Even healthy conditions always have the
potential to change, and illness sets in when meridianal disorders deepen.
Therefore, the development of illness can be prevented by healing a disorder
before it establishes itself in the meridians.

The essence of life is the uninterrupted, continuous beating of the heart
and the action of breathing. The meridians are the pathways for the circulation of *ki*, and the life of the body is maintained by its constant flow. The most
prevalent cause of the stagnation of *ki* are subconscious fears and anxieties
that are manifested as disorders in the mind and body. Even if the causes of
fear and anxiety appear to exist externally, they are in fact merely projected
images of internal feelings. Patients' most prominent preoccupation is the
anxiety that their state of ill health will continue forever. This feeling creates
stress in the sympathetic nerves, which effectively lowers immunity because
the autonomic nerves are closely linked with the functions of immunity. Also, stress in the sympathetic nerves hinders blood flow to the body's periph-
eries, causing muscle contraction. In other words, anxiety about illness
delays recovery. Therefore, in order to promote a speedy recovery from illness, the mind and body must be in a relaxed state, entrusting the disorder
and its cure to nature.

From the classification and name given to specific symptoms, patients
want to know how long their illness will continue. Even healthy people have

a tendency to be particular about anything negative that may be happening to them. For example, some people react angrily to a particular incident and remain in an angry state for a long time afterward, not realizing that what happened to generate their anger already belongs to the past. When this happens, the memory is so strongly fastened to the past incident that the person is unable to react to change. In reality, life exists neither in the past or the future; it exists "here and now"; and when people fixate on an unfavorable incident, they are disturbed by it in the future, which continues to cause stress to the body and mind.

The sage, the ideal in Oriental medicine, is someone who is said to be able to hear the Voice of Nature because he exists "here and now." This ability gives the sage a flexible mind, and he is always able to react to the infinite changes—in other words, to the essence of life. The aim of treatment in Oriental medicine is to release the stagnant *ki* and correct disorders in the mind and body. Through this, the symptoms disappear and the mind, which has become psychologically constrained by prejudices and negativity, can once again become free and flexible.

According to the Eastern ideal, *health* does not simply mean a condition without illness; it is a condition in which the mind and body integrate freely with nature. In Japanese the words once used to mean *health* also meant *flexibility, perfect clarity,* and *not burdened by ego.*[3] Flexibility of mind and body has long been considered of utmost importance to health. Physical flexibility indicates youth: when we are children, our bodies are flexible, but as we grow older, we become increasingly stiff. Flexibility is of primary importance because it enables a range of body movements. For example, if a stick made from hard wood is bent, it will eventually break, but a whip is so flexible that it can bend 360 degrees. In judo, the phrase "flexibility overcomes rigidity" means that true strength is to be found in flexibility and suppleness and not in rigidity. In fact, the word *judo* literally means "the way of flexibility." Flexibility is born in the absence of physical force, because force causes rigidity in the body and diminishes potential physical movement. Flexibility removes the physically defensive attitude toward the outside world and is born

---

3. The Japanese word for health is *kenko.* The first character means health, vigor. It is also pronounced *sukoyaka,* which means total clarity. In Japanese, *sukoyaka* means a clarity of mind not hindered by the ego, in other words, a flexible state. The second character means peace.

from a natural, mental attitude of trust in everything. (Lao-Tzu preached "compliance with nature" and is said to have admired the "flexibility of water.")

It is recognized in clinical psychology that mental tension is equal to muscular tension, and it is possible to say that the strength and freedom of life exist within the flexibility of the mind (yin), which generates flexibility in the body (yang). A Buddhist sutra preaches that "the body and mind of those who bask in Buddha's light soften and generate virtue." Basking in Buddha's light means being liberated from fear and anxiety and developing a mental attitude of entrusting everything to Buddha. The body and mind become flexible, and virtue (the mental search for *satori*— Buddhist enlightenment, nirvana) is born. Zen preaches "detachment from the mind and body," revealing the flexibility of the Buddha Nature. The Buddhist monk Dogen, who preached total detachment from the mind and body and achieved enlightenment, was asked on his return from China what he had learned. He answered simply, "the flexible mind." The flexible mind is none other than wisdom.

When shiatsu therapists are asked what the most important thing is, they are also likely to reply, "the flexible mind." First of all, shiatsu must only be performed by hands that are perfectly flexible and adaptable to any part of the patient's body. Such hands are born from a mind that, through contact with the patient's body, sympathizes with the constant changes in the flow of the natural vital force. In Oriental medicine, diagnosis of the *kyo-jitsu* pattern is also carried out by the flexible mind, which does not halt in any one place. Sustained pressure shiatsu is the expression of the mind entrusted totally to nature. The flexible mind nurtured through this training is one that sympathizes with the *ki* of nature in the patient's body. Sustained pressure shiatsu means being in sympathy with the patient and always becoming passive. Using muscular strength to generate pressure during therapy does not create this fundamental feeling of sympathy with the patient. Also, applying pressure with physical strength results in stress on the patient; even if it is performed in kindness, the patient will remember it as a feeling of oppression. If healers apply pressure without true understanding of their patients' feelings—that is, without sympathy—it is because their ego is standing between them. When there is no understanding, there is no respect and there is no true love. A shiatsu therapy clinic is a place where the individual is respected in the real sense, because the true radiance of life can only be promoted through sympathy, respect, and understanding.

A mistake frequently made by novices performing shiatsu is concentrating their attention on their own fingers and using muscular strength when applying pressure. This type of pressure causes stress in the sympathetic nerves, and the body responds by blocking the stress within the affected area in order to stop it spreading throughout the body. In this case, instead of being liberated, the patient's *ki* is stifled. This is ultimately because the novice healers are directing attention to themselves, disregarding the patients' response to the pressure received. Patients' *ki* is released only when, through shiatsu, they come in contact with the source of their own existence and their response to their own vitality is heightened. This type of shiatsu resounds in the mind, spreads throughout the patients' body, and permeates through to the subconscious. Patients who receive this type of therapy have the potential to return to a state where they are able to grasp the true essence of life. This cannot be achieved by forceful shiatsu where healers are concerned only with themselves as they set out to correct the patient.

The Classics mention "the way of moving *sei* to change *ki*"; in other words, transforming *sei* (the essence of *ki*) causes changes in *ki* (chapter 1). The change in a person's *ki* brought about by shiatsu relieves illness because changes in *ki* change the relationship between the patient and nature and therefore change the patient's way of existing in the natural world. In order to change the patient's *ki*, it is essential not to "change" or "correct" the patient. What the healer can do is be understanding and in sympathy with the patient and read how his or her *ki* responds. Anyone who is told, "That is a bad habit; change it," will only react negatively. Similarly, if healers face patients thinking, "Your body and mind are to blame for this illness, so I'll just fix it for you," they will always encounter unconscious resistance from their patients. The work of the shiatsu therapist is not to correct or change patients but to wholly accept their life through reading their responses to pressure and to allow them the freedom of self-expression. Becoming passive toward patients means accepting their individual existence wholly and not measuring it by other standards. By discarding prejudices and egoistic opinions, healers can face their patients with a clear mind. It is in this mental state that the condition of the patient's life is reflected in the healer's own mind as in a mirror, and diagnosis of the *kyo-jitsu* pattern can take place.

In sustained pressure shiatsu, the healer leaves things entirely up to the patient and is "sustained" or "supported" by the patient, freely entrusting all responses to the patient. This is an expression of faith toward the patient's life offered freely to the healer at time of therapy, and it is an expression of faith toward the patient through a primitive form of message that existed before language. It is transmitted directly through the skin to the lymbic system, the seat of the subconscious (chapter 1). In fact, nothing heightens a person's vital force more than faith in the promise of freedom. What responds to faith is life and there is nothing more valuable to life than freedom. In shiatsu therapy, having faith in the patient's life means having faith in curing the illness through the patient's own vital force. The promise of freedom means that the healer simply and wholly accepts the patient's life, and the patient is allowed the freedom to change or not. In other words, the patient's fundamental being must always be judged favorably and approved of. Life reacts negatively to coercion and responds faithfully to trust; through the guarantee of freedom, it can truly exhibit its fundamental power. Therefore, by receiving the silent message of freedom and faith from the healer through shiatsu, the patient's life is able to regain its original freedom and the patient is released from the handicaps of illness.[4]

In the practice of sustained pressure shiatsu, the healer and patient rely on each other and build a relationship of trust. Then, through the healer, the patient learns to have faith in the power of nature and becomes familiar with the physical sensation of relying on this faith. Through this, the patient's body and mind are released from the closed, fixed state brought on by the caution he or she has until now exercised toward the outside world, and a more profound exchange of *ki* with nature begins. Therefore, the basis of sustained pressure shiatsu is the healer's sympathy toward the patient's life, which is the fundamental spirit of shiatsu. The ideas of sympathizing with and sensing the patient's life cannot be intellectualized. Sympathy does not mean that the healer stands in a high position and reaches down with the hand of salvation to the patient. Rather, the healer and patient each feel the other's actual existence as their own and eventually forget their own existence. When each feels echoes of the other's actual life sensation, they can be likened to the motion of one wave.

A mistake easily made by healers is trying to understand the patient's pain through their own past experiences. Although some would see this as sympathy, it is in fact nothing more than the healers projecting themselves onto the

---

4. The characters for "patient" *(kan-ja)* indicate a person who is pierced through the heart or mind and is unable to move.

patient's condition. In such cases, the healer's mind may easily fixate on the patient's symptoms. What the healer should sympathize with is not the patient's symptoms but the patient's life existing beyond the symptoms, because the patient's life force, not the symptoms, responds to therapy. Through the healer's sympathetic understanding of this, patients are able to recognize the power of life that is the source of their being.

No matter how lonely or distressed we are, we may be healed by someone who is capable of sympathizing with our suffering. In therapy, having sympathy with the patient's life means providing a condition of free exchange between the patient's *ki* and nature. Patients are rescued from their isolation by the intervention of the healer who sympathizes with them and restores them to the original state as one part of the natural world of mutual interrelationships. Rather than actually sympathizing with the patient's suffering, the healer acts as one who can change into light the darkness that lies beneath the surface of that suffering. The essence of life is not sensed through division and contrast but through sympathy and interaction. Each individual's existence may be equated to a tiny island in a vast ocean. In the beginning all these islands were one solid land mass. The notion of sympathy with life in shiatsu therapy is based on the union of the healer and the patient and the feeling that the life of all is one at its source. Union between the healer and the patient is not the joining of the two into one but the loss of boundaries as each comes in contact with the other and both enter a state of nothingness. When the boundaries between ourselves and others are lost, we may feel infinite nothingness without perception of space and time—and feel life as one source: here and now.

In order to acquire this state of sympathy with life in sustained pressure shiatsu, the healer must first of all be open to understanding the patient. He or she must perform treatment while feeling the response of the patient to each application of pressure. The healer must become passive toward the patient and carry out all movements with the purpose of understanding the patient's pre-conscious state of *ki* through which the patient experiences existence as a life indivisible from nature. It is this feeling that heightens the patient's vitality and ultimately guides it toward the healing process.

This sympathy with life does not exist only in shiatsu therapy. Sympathy and a close connection with others should be fundamental to all human relations. However, modern times have brought about a disintegration into illness. Recently, sympathy and contact between people have weakened, and as we become more self-centered, our main concerns are individualism and isolationism. Our relationship with nature has also weakened, and we have lost focus on our bodies, our closest connection with nature.

When we receive shiatsu, which can also be performed among friends and family, daily, we become sensitive to the natural messages from our body and our body, rather than our head, becomes the subject. Our body is revitalized, enabling us to begin a more justifiable existence. When this happens, we are no longer able to sustain the compulsive lifestyle of business and enterprise. We may reach the point where we can only live simply and candidly, without wishing to acquire more fame and position than those around us. The happiness and well-being we acquire means liberation from the prosaic earthly mind that compares ourselves to others. Sustained pressure shiatsu is no more than the experience of a life that does not distinguish between the self and others and the recognition of the world of incomparable *ki*.

Continuous Steady Pressure

Maintaining continuous pressure means that the healer's body remains in an absolutely "still" state, so that even, constant pressure can be applied to the patient's body for a given period of time. Masunaga claims that the use of continuous and steady pressure is the main difference between shiatsu therapy and other manual healing techniques such as massage. When continuous, steady pressure is applied to the body, the patient's sensation of being separate from the healer dulls and the primal sense as well as actual feelings of life are aroused within the patient. It is not possible to maintain constant pressure if it is applied with physical strength. If the same degree of pressure is not maintained for a specific period of time, the body is unable to remain in a totally relaxed state, which means that it is unable to be awakened to the primal sensations. In shiatsu, it is possible to influence the whole body by applying pressure to only one point. However, if the pressure is applied for too short a time, it only affects a limited part of the body. The applied pressure must induce changes throughout the patient's body. (This reflects the Eastern perception that the part is to be found in the whole and the whole in the part.)

Shiatsu does not heal through the application of physical pressure. If the shiatsu healer were able to cure an illness through physical pressure, there would be little difference from the Western practice of artificial manipulation of the physical body. The application of pressure in shiatsu therapy influences the whole body and allows the patient's *ki* to collect within his or her body. Physically maintaining steady pressure may be illustrated by the example of the way in which people stand up. When people stand naturally, the soles of their feet carry the entire pressure of the body. This is a continuous pressure similar to the pressure at the point of contact of the healer's body weight on the patient's body.

Healers must be careful not to use only the weight of the top half of their body when leaning on the patient, because doing so will gradually exhaust their own *ki*. This is because the weight of the top part of the body and that of the lower part of the body are separate, and when applying pressure the movement of the body must work as a whole. It is best to lean with the upper part of the body while visualizing leaning with the weight of the lower part of the body. By doing this, the healer's whole body weight is in contact with the patient, enabling the appropriate application of steady, continuous pressure and ensuring that the healer's *ki* is not exhausted.

Using Precisely the Same Pressure on Four Points

Since the healer uses both arms and legs to exert pressure, there are two points of contact with the patient and two points of contact with the ground, and the application of pressure is the same on all four points (Figure 2.14). This does not mean that the total pressure is divided by four and that a quarter is applied to each of the four points of contact. The healer's arms and legs each use a hundred percent of the whole body weight. When shiatsu is performed with this image, patients lose the sensation of boundaries between themselves and their healer and a mutual current of *ki* flows freely between them. At this point patients are no longer able to feel which part of their body is being touched, their sense of discrimination is dulled, and their primal sense is aroused. When patients no longer feel they exist as a separate entity, they sense the *ki* in their entire body. At this point, the healer's conscious recognition of space and time becomes blurred and he or she senses an incomparably vast space.

Distribution of the Healer's Body Weight

Explained in practical terms, when the patient is lying face down and the healer exerts pressure with the palms of his or her hands, the weight of the

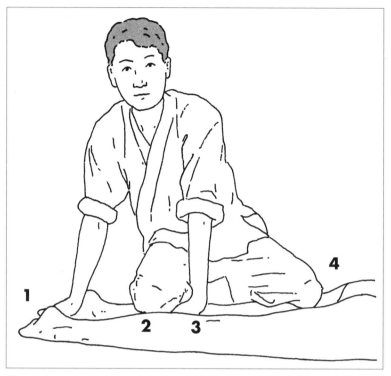

Figure 2.14

healer's lower part of the body is deliberately transferred to the upper part and to the hands. The pressure created by the body weight needs to exist in a perfect balance between the lower part of the healer's body and the healer's hands. In this position, healers are able to maintain the exact amount of equal pressure and their *ki* is also able to flow through the patient's body. With each application of pressure, healers must carefully observe the position of their own body to ensure that they do not lean too far forward or backward. Their body must be maintained at a perfect balance similar to that of a Japanese balancing toy, which perches on a tiny point by means of two weights hanging from its long arms.

The Absolute Steadiness of the Healer's Body

What is most important in maintaining steady pressure is the stability of the healer's body. A simple test is to push the healer from the side while he or she is applying pressure to a patient lying down to see if balance is lost. If balance is lost, it means that constant pressure was not being applied. When the healer's *ki* is faithfully passing through to the patient, however hard one pushes the healer, he or she will remain in a stable position. The reason the healer does not fall is that the healer visualizes his or her body being perfectly stable. Using this technique, the healer is in a relaxed state, with *ki* passing freely through to the patient, making it difficult to lose balance even when pushed from the side. This state is easily achieved through visualizing both the hands (the points of contact with the patient) and the knees or feet (the points of contact with the earth) at the same level, without awareness of the difference in height of each. (The technique is very simple and I encourage you to try it.) If the image is maintained, the healer is very stable and does not lose balance when pushed. However, as soon as this image is interrupted he or she can be pushed over easily. See Figure 2.15.

The following experiment also uses the visualization technique. This time it is not the healer who visualizes the hands and knees at the same level, but a third person nearby. The third person does not touch the healer or the patient at any time but holds in his or her mind a very strong image that the healer's "hands and knees are at the same level." When a third person visualizes this, a fourth person cannot make the healer lose balance, even by pushing forcefully. (Note that the fourth person is not the visualizer.) This phenomenon occurs because *ki* follows what is essentially understood to be visualization.

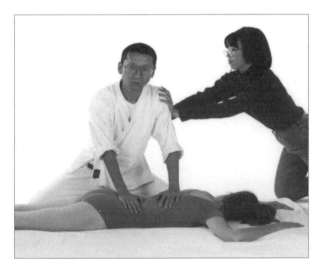

Figure 2.15

These experiments show that the discipline of shiatsu is image training rather than technical training (chapter 1). Furthermore, one is able to feel the actual force and power working on the body of the person holding the image. In the experiments mentioned above, the potential of the image to function even through a third person is reminiscent of the power of prayer.

Perpendicular Pressure

Perpendicular pressure is usually described as pressure applied vertically to the surface of the body, but I want to offer a new perspective on this based on the principle of *ki*. I feel a new interpretation of perpendicular pressure is necessary because the body surface is not flat, and the real meaning of this technique involves more than has been previously understood. I believe perpendicular pressure should mean that the healer's arms are perpendicular to the patient's spine rather than perpendicular to the body surface. In most shiatsu techniques, when one applies continuous steady pressure, the arms are in an extended position, therefore at a right angle to the spine. A better explanation of the spine is the line joined by the three points of the upper *tanden*, central *tanden*, and lower *tanden*: in other words, the Conception Vessel (see Figure 2.16).

The upper *tanden* is the point in the middle of the forehead. In Buddhist images a dot is painted on this point. In yoga this point is considered to be of utmost importance because it is where one focuses awareness during meditation. The central *tanden* is in the center of the breastbone and what is called the chest line in kinetology, a function-

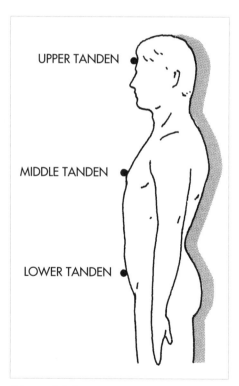

UPPER TANDEN

MIDDLE TANDEN

LOWER TANDEN

Figure 2.16

al study of the practical use of movement. According to George Guthart, its founder, kinetology regards the chest line to be the "seam" between the mind and body and its role is to control the immune function and the self-healing strength generated by the life force. The lower *tanden*, usually simply called the *tanden*, is about five to nine centimeters below the navel and is the center of *ki*. All the classical arts in Japan, from the tea ceremony to Noh, use this point as the center of concentration from which every movement originates.

Perpendicular pressure is applied with straight arms perpendicular to the three *tanden*. Both the neck and back must be straight, as in the sitting position in Zen meditation. A common mistake among beginners is to look at one's hands while applying pressure. It is important to remember that because there is a strong connection between the line of vision and *ki*, if the healer looks at his or her own hands (even for a short moment), the flow of *ki* will stop. Also, the healer should not bend his or her head toward the hands during shiatsu practice because this exhausts *ki*.

The Principles of the *Ki* Shiatsu Method

Theory and Techniques of the *Ki* Shiatsu Method

The *ki* shiatsu method is the most recent and most advanced shiatsu technique to be developed. Previously, a form of shiatsu therapy had originated in Japan in the Taisho period (1912–1926) that was initially a mainstream version of a form of therapy using finger pressure to relieve stiffness in parts of the body through the strength of one's muscles. Professional healers emerged everywhere and, particularly if they were able to discharge strong *ki* despite not knowing the theory of meridians, cured illness through the power of *ki* and gained people's confidence. It is said that some healers professed to be able to cure cancer and advertised in the media that they had proof of having cured government officials. Such healers existed all over Japan but did not have the theoretical background to hand down their technique, so the technique did not survive past their own generation. Techniques such as the *ki* shiatsu method, however, are both theoretically and practically advanced, and have been able to be handed down through successive generations.

It was Shizuto Masunaga who argued that shiatsu was not to be performed through physical pressure (the pressure of the healer's body weight), as had been the case in the Taisho period, but that it was now to be performed using sustained pressure, on the basis of which he then developed the new technique of channeling the patient's *ki*. When this technique reached the standard of *ki* shiatsu method, the previous methods of physical application of pressure to the patient's body became obsolete. This basic technique of *ki* shiatsu channels *ki* by moving the patient's skin. This is known as applying pressure by "taking up the slack of the skin" (see Figure 2.17). By acquiring knowledge of this technique, healers are able not only to cure illness and stimulate a holistic response in their patients but also to heighten their own *ki*.

I attended a series of lectures on macrobiotics (a method of health maintenance through diet) in which Hideo Oomori explained that macrobiotics categorizes all food into yin and yang. He suggested that time could be expressed as alternating yin and yang periods of about eight hundred years each. The yang period is one of material innovation, and because it is a period of male domination in society, there is constant conflict. In Japan it was just eight hundred years ago when the rise of war-favoring samurai suppressed the lifestyles of pleasure through the arts and performances of the nobility. According to Oomori, that particular yang period ended around 1945 with World War II, and we are now entering a yin period. A yin period fosters spiritualism instead of materialism. It is said to be a period of feminine harmony rather than masculine conflict, of sensitivity rather than reason, of religion and the arts rather than political ideology. He suggested that altruism based on a spiritual culture will emerge from the materialist civilizations existing until now. Furthermore, the yang energy, such as the energy of coal and oil used until now, will be replaced by an abundance of yin energy, such as hydrogen produced from the waters of the ocean.[5]

From my own experience in shiatsu therapy throughout the years, I have noticed a marked increase in patients with the *kyo* pattern in the meridians (a yin complaint). In Masunaga's days (1955–1985) most patients presented the *jitsu* pattern (a yang complaint), and those who presented the *kyo* pattern

---

5.   Hideo Oomori, lecture at Tokyo Macrobiotic Center, July 1982.

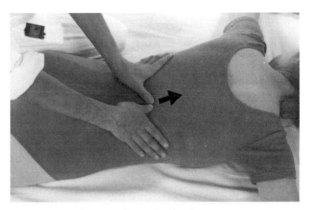

Figure 2.17a.   Touching the body

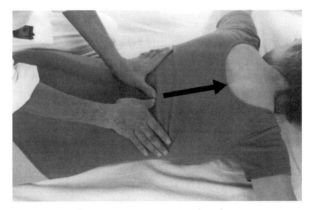

Figure 2.17b.   Starting to move the skin

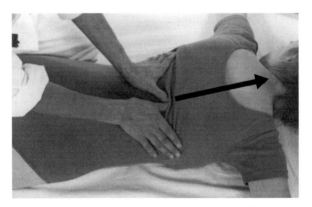

Figure 2.17c.   Moving skin to the physical limit

belonged to a group of people suffering from chronic diseases. *Kyosho* patients began to increase around the mid to late 1980s and at present these constitute around 90 percent of all complaints.

I began to wonder if this phenomenon were due to increasing dependence on intoxicating drugs. But even so, there were far too many patients with *kyo* stiffness and pain. Furthermore, these complaints of stiffness and pain caused by the *kyo* pattern were not easily relieved by the *sha* method. For instance, in acupuncture, if chronic *kyo* pain or stiffness is treated with a strong *sha* needle, it may result in the patient's being unable to stand up the following day. In order to safeguard against such unfavorable effects, there must always be precise distinction between the *ho* and *sha* needles and it is necessary to always carry out *ho* therapy on the *kyo* condition. This means that it is extremely dangerous to perform needle therapy with disregard to the state of the meridians.

The current prevalence of the *kyo* pattern may indicate that the yin era has begun. As we enter a yin era, the medical techniques suitable for treating symptoms of the materialistic, aggressive yang nature are no longer effective. Therefore there is a need to change from yang medicine based on the body to a more spiritual yin medicine based on the functions of *ki* and the mind.

Based on this concept of yin and yang periods of time, we may arrive at an explanation for why needles, which were mainstream in Chinese medicine until recent years, have been replaced by disciplines such as *qigong*. In other words, *sha* therapy through the use of needles has been replaced by *ho* therapy through emphasis on methods of healing that do not focus on tools. Shiatsu therapy, which developed from the previous yang technique of using physical strength, has also shifted to the yin technique of channeling the patient's *ki* without the use of physical strength. Astrologically, the present change from a period of yang to a period of yin is expected to affect the change from the Pisces age to the spiritual age of Aquarius at the end of the twentieth century. It is thought that people will awaken to an era of spirituality (meaning that the individual's spiritual nature will be heightened). Art and medicine too will change from the methods of physical science to a focus on spirituality. As such, shiatsu must also develop methods suitable for the spiritual yin era. With this as its background, shiatsu therapy, as the medical study of meridians, will inevitably hold a prominent place as the medicine of *ki* that integrates yin and yang.

Directing *Ki* by Taking up the Slack of the Skin

Applying pressure in order to direct *ki* is characteristic of the *ki* shiatsu method. This is one of the techniques used in aikido to control the other person's mind and body. Directing *ki* is a common aspect of the *ki* shiatsu method and the martial arts, suggesting what may be an ideal technique of basic shiatsu. This is because the method of training one's own *ki* in martial arts is identical to that in the shiatsu method, and through repeated shiatsu therapy on others, the healer gains the benefits of enriching his or her own *ki*.

It is possible to channel *ki* using the technique of taking up the slack of the skin because when the skin is moved, the whole body moves. The "whole body" also includes the mind, and *ki* is channeled not by touching one part of the body but by having whole body "move at the same time." In other words, *ki* is channeled through the relaxation of the whole surface of the patient's body through touch. The *ki* shiatsu method is not based on manipulation of the patient's body by the healer. The object of therapy in *ki* shiatsu is the body of *ki*, which is invisible to the naked eye.

Rudolf Steiner proposes that apart from the physical body, humans have five bodies, two of which are the ether body and the astral body. The astral body in particular controls the flow of energy by following certain lines. When there is emotional distress, this flow of energy stagnates, causing physical ailment.[6] The *ki* shiatsu method does not focus on pressing the patient's body, nor on stimulating biological functions. It does, however, touch the body of *ki* and by doing so cures physical illness because the physical body is like the shadow of the much more powerful body of *ki*.

But when the healer takes up the slack of the skin, where is *ki* channeled to? The answer is one and a half meters beyond the place where the slack of the skin is taken up. One and a half meters is specified here because the size of the body of *ki* is about a one-and-a-half-meter radius. The healer applies pressure by taking up the slack of the patient's skin and when a certain limit has been reached, the healer's body enters a state of repose (which is not to be mistaken for a state of fixation). While the healer's body is physically immobile, his or her *ki* continues to be projected one and a half meters ahead.

---

6. Considering this, one wonders whether the "certain lines" flowing in the ether body are not the meridians and the ether body itself is not the body of *ki*.

The Direction of *Ki* and the Movement of the Healer's Body

The angle at which the healer directs *ki* is always the direction in which the patient's skin moves most naturally when pressed. The healer must take great care in this because the correct angle cannot be found if body weight is applied. In moving the fingers, the healer must not neglect the fact that the source of the movement is in his or her whole body. Therefore, the movement of the fingers that take up slack and the movement of the healer's body must be in perfect union from beginning to end. There are some students who continue to move their body even after the *ki* has been directed (this happens when body weight is applied). However, such unnecessary body movement in this technique in fact weakens the function of *ki*.

Furthermore, when giving shiatsu in order to direct *ki*, the healer's body is physically in a state of rest. However, this differs from mere immobility; it is more like the state of the bow just before the arrow is released. In other words, the healer's body and concentration always continue to be focused ahead beyond the patient. At such times, even though the healer's body is not moving physically, his or her energy continues to be projected forward.

Directing *Ki* to the Deepest Level

All application of pressure in the *ki* shiatsu method may be performed correctly through the use of the Conception Vessel in the arms, the *tanden*, and the Governor Vessel in the legs. The Conception Vessel in the arms runs between the ring finger and the little finger (between the Heart and Liver Meridians), and the Governor Vessel in the legs runs along the Kidney Meridian. Previous diagrams of meridians did not note these vessels in the arms and legs. In using these vessels and meridians, the healer first of all locates the Conception Vessel in the arms and directs *ki* by taking up the slack of the skin superficially. (At this time the lower half of the healer's body is the central point of the movement.) Then, through the process of deepening the technique of channeling *ki* toward the center of the body, the healer's awareness is transferred from the *tanden* to the Governor Vessel in the legs (the focal point of this movement is in the upper half of the healer's body). Therefore, when the healer channels *ki* to reach the center of the patient's body, the energy (the patient's response to pressure) flows from the healer's Conception Vessel in the arms to his or her *tanden*, and then to the Governor Vessel.

Applying pressure in order to direct *ki* to the center of the body is not only carried out through the *sha* technique of applying pressure by using the fingers, hands, knees, and so on. Similarly, the *ho* technique (the supporting hand) is not simply used on the surface of the body. These techniques must direct *ki* to the center of the body, at which time, a mysterious feeling is stimulated within the patient because the focal point of the direction of *ki* of the *ho* technique and that of the *sha* technique become one. The center of the body to which *ki* penetrates is, in fact, the center of the body of *ki*, which surpasses physical dimensions as it unites the focal points of the *ho* and *sha* techniques. Taking up slack in order to direct *ki* toward the center of the body may be expressed as something very similar to "moving the flesh away from the bones."

These are the three principles of the *ki* shiatsu method. They are not methods of physical manipulation but of visualization. In other words, the *ki* shiatsu method involves the stimulation of the patient's body of *ki* by the healer's body of *ki*. Mastering the *ki* shiatsu method strengthens the healer's powers of visualization, which enrich his or her own *ki* and strengthen the *tanden*. The ancient Chinese practices of *doin-ankyo* noted in the Classics are methods of enriching one's vitality by channeling *ki*. The shiatsu healing techniques based on the *ki* shiatsu method may be traced back to the essence of *doin-ankyo*, which makes shiatsu become the center of Oriental medical practices.

Furthermore, pressure application in the *ki* shiatsu method may be the same in both *ho* and *sha* or it may differ. In each technique, the direction of taking up slack is explained in the next section, The Basic Forms of Tao Shiatsu; the direction of *ho* is indicated by the broken line, and *sha* by the unbroken line.

The Basic Forms of Tao Shiatsu

The basic techniques of whole-body shiatsu are practiced on the patient lying in one of three positions: on the side, face down, or face up (the latter includes sitting). Shiatsu is generally practiced first with the patient lying on his or her side, and then with the patient face down. Then, the patient lies on his or her back, and the healer performs *hara* diagnosis, follows with meridianal treatment according to meridianal diagnosis, and concludes with treatment to the *hara* region. All these basic procedures have a clinical significance on which they are structured. Here, I would like to explain simply the procedures in each position of the body.

Lying on Side

The shiatsu performed on the patient lying on the side begins with treatment of the legs. This is because the healer can bring the patient's *ki* down by performing treatment on the legs, which will, to a certain extent, soften any stiffness that may be present in the upper body as well, facilitating treatment there. This is particularly true for stiffness and pain caused by the *jitsu* pattern, because it is generated by the accumulation of *ki* and may be relieved by the dissipation of *ki*. Naturally, treatment is not complete until meridianal therapy has been carried out, but beginning with shiatsu on the legs has the advantage of avoiding the so-called return of stiffness that sometimes happens on the day after treatment.

Shiatsu performed on patients in this position is the most important of all the basic forms. Also, after finishing the basic forms of shiatsu, the healer performs meridianal diagnosis, which may heighten the effects of the treatment. Shiatsu techniques for this position can also be performed on pregnant women.

Lying Face Down

Shiatsu performed with the patient lying face down heightens the effect of the basic shiatsu techniques performed on the patient lying on the side. This includes applying palm pressure to the arms, elbow pressure to the back and hips, and pressure on the legs.

Lying Face Up

Before learning the techniques of diagnosing the *kyo-jitsu* pattern and those of shiatsu therapy, the healer begins by carrying out basic shiatsu with the patient lying face up. Because this position includes the basic forms of meridianal therapy on the limbs and touch diagnosis of the *hara* area (four finger shiatsu on the *hara* area), healers who begin by learning these techniques will find other forms of meridianal treatment to be more easily acquired.

Lying on Side

Begin with the patient on his or her right side and the healer behind the patient.

1. Grasping pressure to the left thigh area

Ho: Place your left hand on the patient's left foot.

Sha: Apply grasping pressure to the patient's thigh with the whole of your right hand. Repeat twice on three points.

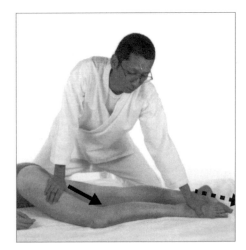

1. Grasping pressure to thigh

2. Thumb pressure to the left leg

Grasp the calf and place both thumbs evenly on the back of the lower leg. Apply pressure to the calf while rotating backward by taking up the slack of the skin. The pressure is applied evenly through the fingers and thumbs of both hands. Repeat twice on three points.

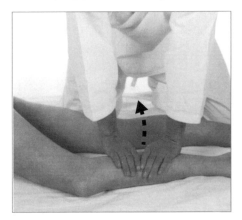

2. Thumb pressure to leg

3. Clipping pressure to the outside of the left foot

Ho: Place your right hand on the patient's ankle.

Sha: Hold the patient's foot between the thumb and the four fingers with the thumb on the top

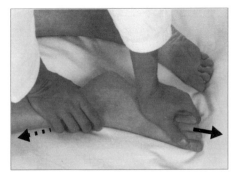

3. Clipping pressure to foot

of the foot. Apply clipping pressure on three points toward the heel. Repeat twice.

4. Knee pressure to the right inner thigh area

Ho: Place your left hand on the bottom of the patient's right foot and right hand on the patient's buttock.

Sha: Apply pressure to the patient's inner thigh area with the right knee. Repeat twice on three points.

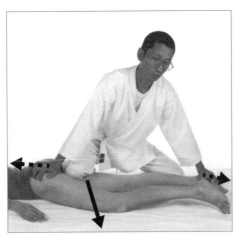

4. Knee pressure to thigh

5. Left knee pressure to the lower right leg

Ho: With your left hand on the bottom of the patient's right foot and your right hand on the patient's upper right calf, place your right knee against the patient's inner thigh, close to the crotch.

Sha: Apply left knee pressure to the patient's lower leg. Repeat twice on three points toward the ankle.

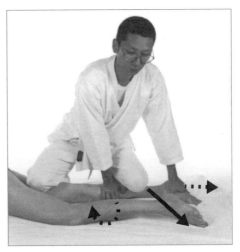

5. Left knee pressure to lower leg

6. Left knee pressure to the bottom of the right foot

Ho: Hold the patient's ankle with your right hand and place your left hand on the floor.

Sha: Apply left knee pressure from the arch of the foot toward the tips

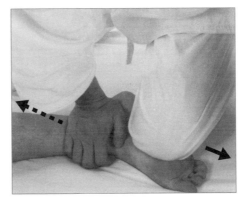

6. Left knee pressure to foot

of the toes. Repeat twice on three points.

7. Heel of the hand pressure to the side of the head

Posture: Place yourself parallel to the patient. Raise your right knee and place the side of your left thigh against the patient's upper back.

Ho: Place your left palm on the patient's temple.

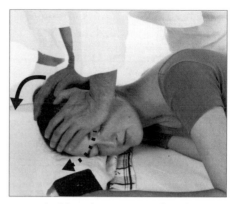

7. Heel of hand pressure to head

Sha: Apply pressure to the side of the patient's head with the heel of your right hand. Repeat twice on three points toward the neck.

8. Left palm pressure to the side of the face

Ho: Place your right palm on the side of the patient's head.

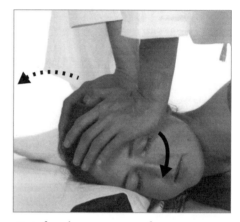

8. Left palm pressure to face

Sha: With your left palm apply pressure from the temple to the jawbone. Repeat twice on three points.

9. Grasping pressure with the thumb on the neck

Ho: Place your left hand on the patient's shoulder joint, and feel the patient's body rising as you press.

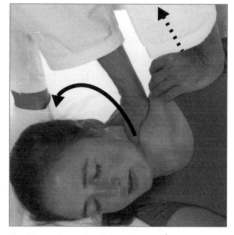

9. Grasping pressure on neck

Sha: Grasp the neck area with the whole of your right hand and thumb. Apply pressure by rotating while taking up slack three times on each of three lines: the front, side, and back of the neck.

10. Ulna pressure to the neck

Posture: With your left thigh against the patient's back, bring your right knee down to line up with the left.

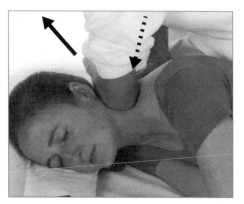

10. Ulna pressure to neck

Ho: Place your right palm on the patient's spine. Press down toward the floor.

Sha: The left ulna is parallel with the floor. Apply ulna pressure to three points on the neck region.

11. Ulna pressure to the upper point of the shoulder blade

Posture: Kneel at the head of the patient, with the balls of your feet on the floor.

Ho: Place your left palm on the patient's upper spine.

Sha: Apply right ulna pressure to the upper joint of the shoulder blade on three points, starting from the shoulder. Repeat twice.

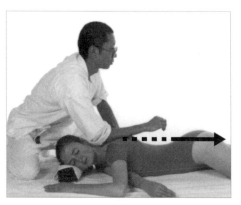

11. Ulna pressure to shoulder

12. Pressure of both thumbs to the left side of the spine

A. *Posture:* Kneel, perpendicular to the patient, with the balls of your feet on the floor.

Apply pressure from the shoulders down to the lower back with both thumbs evenly placed and supported by the four fingers of both hands.

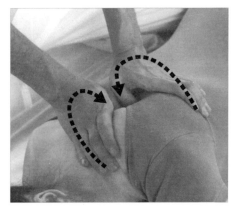

12 A. Thumb pressure to upper spine

B. *Posture:* Change posture at around the tenth thoracic vertebrae; place yourself parallel to the patient.

Apply pressure with both thumbs down to the sacral bone. (The angle of each thumb to the spinal column is about 45 degrees.)

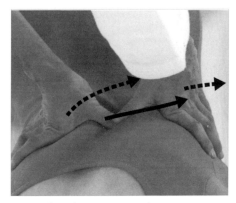

12 B. Thumb pressure to lower spine

C. Pressure of both thumbs to the inner shoulder blade

Posture: Return to the posture in A.

Apply pressure with both thumbs to the inner shoulder blade. Repeat A, B, and C in sequence.

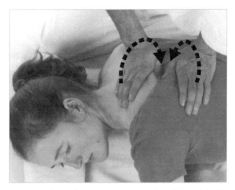

12 C. Thumb pressure to shoulder blade

13. Ulna pressure to the left arm

Posture: Resting on the balls of your feet, raise both knees and place them lightly against the patient's side.

Ho: Place the patient's left arm on your knees and hold the wrist with your left hand.

Sha: With your right ulna, apply pressure to three points each on the patient's upper and lower arm, moving down toward the tips of the fingers. Repeat twice.

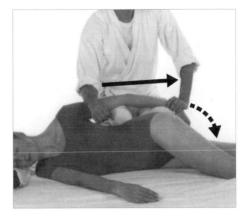

13. Ulna pressure to arm

14. Grasping pressure to the arm

A. *Ho:* Bend the patient's arm and place the back of the hand on the side of the patient's waist. Grasp the wrist with your left hand.

   Sha: Apply grasping pressure to three points of the upper arm with your right hand, taking up slack while rotating backwards.

B. *Ho:* Keep your right hand on the last point of pressure on the upper arm.

   Sha: Apply grasping pressure to three points of the forearm with the left hand from the elbow to the wrist.

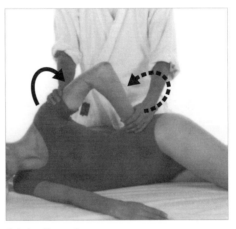

14 A. Grasping pressure to upper arm

Repeat A and B twice.

15. Moving the arms

Posture: Place yourself parallel to
the patient, with your left thigh
against the patient's back.

Ho: Place your right hand on top of
the shoulder, making this the pivot.

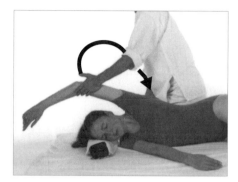

15. Moving the arms

Sha: Cup the inside of the patient's
elbow with your left hand and
rotate the patient's arm. Repeat
three times.

16. Ulna pressure to the inside of
the patient's upper arm

Ho: On the last rotation from step
15, leave the patient's arm resting
against the side of his or her head
and place your right hand on the
patient's elbow.

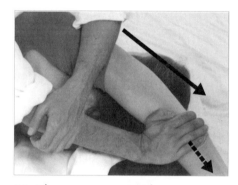

Sha: Apply left ulna pressure from
just below the shoulder bone to
the elbow and from the inside of
the upper arm to the elbow.

16. Ulna pressure to inside arm

17. Arm extension

Posture: Place yourself perpendicular to the patient and raise your hips.

A. Your right hand is on the patient's elbow and your left hand is on the hip. While leaning with your body weight, spread your arms to left and right. Once only.

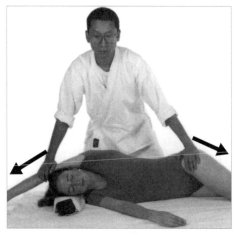

17 A. Hands on elbow and hip

B. Take the patient's left wrist and hold tightly in both hands with interlaced fingers. Pull the arm toward your own chest, and then let your own body lean backward slightly. After having extended the arm, drop it gently. Once only.

18. Ulna pressure to the left side of the back

Posture: Place yourself parallel to the patient, with the outside of your left thigh against the patient's back and your right knee raised.

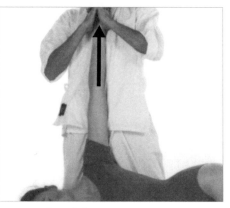

17 B. Pulling left wrist

Ho: The right palm follows the right *sha* elbow and moves with it simultaneously.

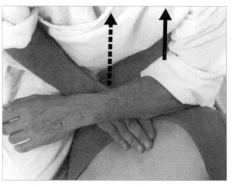

18. Ulna pressure to back

Sha: With the left ulna, apply pressure on several points from the lower part of the shoulder blade down to the waist. Then apply pressure on several points from the waist down to the buttocks.

19. Elbow pressure to (A) the side of the spinal column and (B) the inner side of the shoulder blade

Posture: Place yourself perpendicular to the patient.

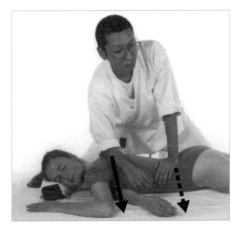

19. Pressure to spine and shoulder

Ho: Place your left hand on the side of the patient's waist.

Sha: A. With the right elbow, apply pressure to several points on the side of spinal column from the shoulder blade to around the middle of the back. *B.* In the same way, apply elbow pressure to the inner side of the shoulder blade on four points. Repeat A and B twice.

20. Right elbow pressure to the lower back

Posture: Slide yourself lower toward the patient's hips.

Ho: Place your left ulna on the patient's hips.

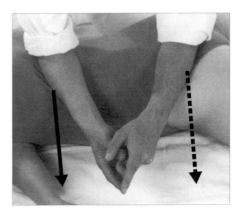

20. Elbow pressure to lower back

Sha: Apply right elbow pressure to several points on the side of the spine, beginning at the lower back and continuing to the upper sacrum.

21. Left knee pressure to the back of the thigh

Posture: Place your left knee in a perpendicular position to the thigh that is to receive the pressure.

Ho: Place your right elbow on the patient's hip. Your left hand is on the upper part of the lower leg.

Sha: Apply left knee pressure to the back of the upper leg on three points. Repeat twice.

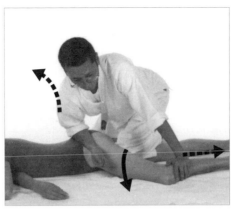

21. Knee pressure to thigh

22. Pressure of both thumbs on the outside of the lower left leg

Posture: Drop both knees and raise your hips.

Ho: Place your fingers on the back of the patient's lower leg. Position both thumbs evenly on the outside of the lower leg.

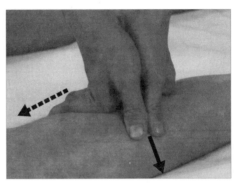

22. Thumb pressure to lower leg

Sha: Press by taking up slack toward the floor on three points down the leg. Repeat twice.

23. Clipping pressure and expansion of the outside of the foot

Ho: Place your right hand on the patient's ankle.

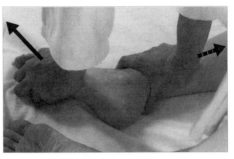

23. Clipping pressure to foot

Sha: Apply clipping pressure with the thumb and four fingers. Repeat twice on three points. Then, with the heel of the left hand, apply pressure toward the tips of the toes while stretching the area.

24. Knee pressure to right thigh, lower leg, and bottom of foot

Same as steps 4, 5, and 6.

25. Spinal twist

Posture: Place yourself perpendicular to the patient and raise your hips.

Place your right hand on the front of the left shoulder area near the underarm. Apply pressure by pushing the left shoulder toward the floor. Place your left hand on the patient's lower left thigh, taking up slack in the direction opposite to the right hand.

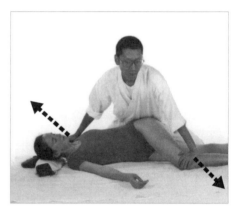

25. Spinal twist

26. Stretching the side of the body

With your right hand, apply pressure to the patient's left shoulder blade. Place your left knee against the back of the upper thigh near the buttock, making this the pivot. Place your left hand on the front of lower thigh and pull as though to draw the leg closer by taking up slack in the direction opposite to the right hand.

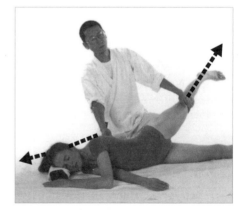

26. Stretching side of body

27.Completion

Ho: Place your left hand on the patient's lower back.

Sha: Apply palm pressure on three points on the side of the spine, taking up slack toward the feet with both hands simultaneously and in the same direction. Once only. Then lightly brush off *ki* with a downward movement using the right hand from the shoulders to the buttocks. Repeat twice.

Repeat steps 1–27 on the patient's opposite side.

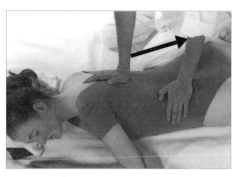

27. Completion

Lying Face Down

1. Walking the hands on the patient's arms and back

Apply pressure using your whole hands with a "walking" motion from the shoulder blade down the arms to the hands and back to the shoulder blade. Then, walk your hands from the shoulder blade to the sacral bone and back to the shoulder blade.

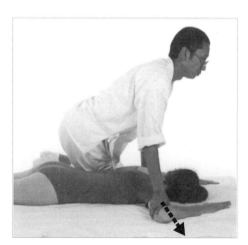

1. Walking the hands on arms and back

2. Elbow pressure to the upper
   back and sides of spine

Posture: Kneel on your left knee
and place your right knee at the
patient's armpit, resting on your
right foot.

Ho: With your left hand, grasp the
middle of the patient's left upper
arm.

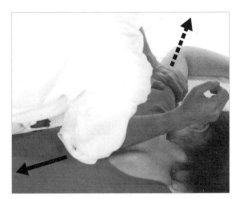

2. Elbow pressure to upper back

Sha: Apply right elbow pressure on
several points on the left side of the
spine in the upper back, then on
the right side of the spine.

3. Elbow pressure to the lower back

Posture: Slide down to the lower
part of the patient's body. Place
your left palm on the patient's
spine.

Ho: Place your right elbow
between index finger and thumb
of your left hand.

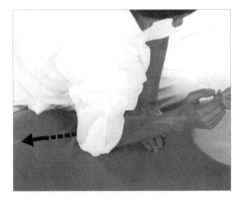

3. Elbow pressure to lower back

Sha: Apply pressure with left hand
and right elbow together, on both
sides of the spine at several points
from the lower back area to the
waist. Then from the sacral area to
the buttocks, taking up slack
toward the head. Once on each side
on several points.

4. One-point knee pressure to the buttocks

Posture: Place yourself perpendicular to the patient.

Place your left kneecap on the deepest point of the patient's left buttock, and with both hands draw the right hip bone upward and toward you. Hold for two to three seconds.

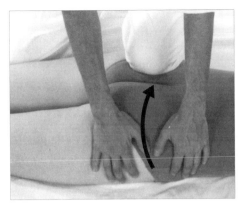

4. One-point knee pressure to buttocks

5. Knee pressure to the left thigh

Ho: Keeping your left knee on the patient's buttocks, place your left palm on the sacral bone area. Grasp the patient's ankle with your right hand and raise the lower leg.

Sha: With your right knee, apply knee pressure on three points along each of the three lines from the inside of the thigh to the back of the thigh.

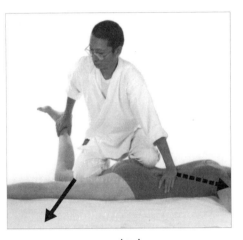

5. Knee pressure to thigh

6. Knee pressure to the lower leg

Posture: Return the patient's raised lower leg to the ground.

Ho: Place your left knee on the back of the patient's thigh where it meets the buttock. Place your left hand and right knee on the lower leg and move your right hand to the bottom of the foot.

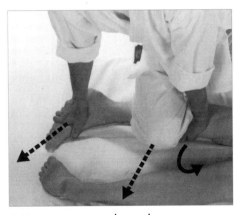

6. Knee pressure to lower leg

Sha: Lean forward (parallel with the floor) and apply pressure with your left hand (*sha*) and right knee (*ho*) without using your body weight. Repeat twice on three points toward the heel.

7. Right knee pressure to the sole of the foot

Ho: Put your right hand on the floor and grasp the ankle with your left hand.

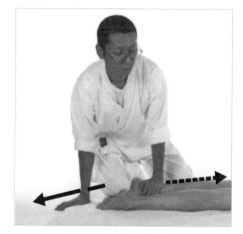

7. Knee pressure to sole of foot

Sha: With your right knee, apply pressure on three points toward the tips of the toes. Repeat twice.

Move to the patient's right side and repeat steps 1–7.

8. Leg extension

A. Grasp the outside of both feet and bend the lower legs up toward the head. Stretch to the tips of the toes by taking up the slack of the skin.

B. Now hold the bottom of the feet and flex the toes toward the floor directing *ki* toward the tips of the toes (not shown in photo).

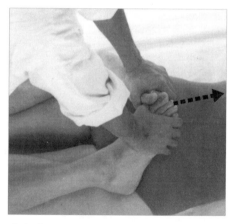

8 A. Leg extension

9. Extension pressure to the outside of the leg

Posture: Move the patient's left thigh out to a right angle with the body.

Ho: Place your right knee on the bottom of the patient's left foot and your left hand on the patient's buttock.

Sha: With your right palm take up slack on four points on the outside of the leg. Repeat twice on each leg.

10. *Seiza* sitting pressure on thighs

Sit quietly on the patient's thigh area without applying force.

11. Standing pressure on the soles of the feet

Facing the patient, stand up and place the heels of your feet in the arches of the patient's feet.

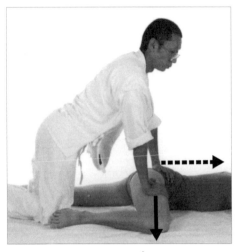

9. Extension pressure to leg

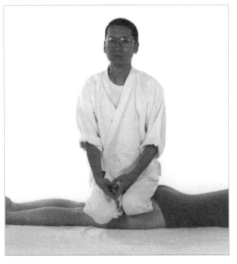

10. *Seiza* sitting pressure on thighs

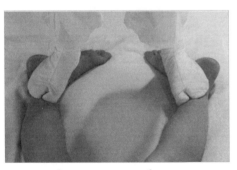

11. Standing pressure on feet

12. Completion on the legs

Ho: Place both your knees on the soles of the patient's feet.

Sha: Apply pressure with both palms on four points on the thigh and lower leg. Repeat twice.

13. Completion on the back area

A. Place both palms on the shoulder blade and apply palm pressure in a circular motion rotating inward.

B. Place both palms on the hip area and take up the slack of the skin by moving up and down.

C. Place both palms on the buttocks and apply pressure with the heels of the hands in a circular motion rotating outward.

D. Stimulate the flow of *ki* by crossing your palms one on top of the other and placing them on the patient's spine, then brushing up and down the spine lightly and quickly. Repeat twice.

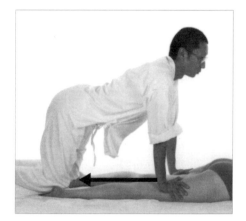

12. Completion on legs

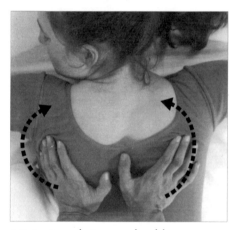

13 A. Completion on shoulder area

Lying Face Up and Sitting

1. *Hara* diagnosis

Posture: Sit in *seiza* (or on your heels with the balls of your feet on the floor) on the patient's left side. Place your left hand on your knees.

Ho: Place your right thigh alongside the patient's hip.

Sha: Perform *hara* diagnosis with the four fingers of the right hand.

2. Heel of the hand pressure to the inside of the leg (Small Intestine Meridian)

Posture: Place yourself perpendicular to the patient. The patient's knee is bent at a right angle.

Ho: Place your left hand on the patient's *hara*.

Sha: Apply pressure of the hand twice on each of three points on the left thigh and lower leg. Repeat on the right thigh and lower leg.

3. Ulna pressure to the outside of the leg (Triple Heater Meridian)

Ho: Place your left hand on the patient's *hara*.

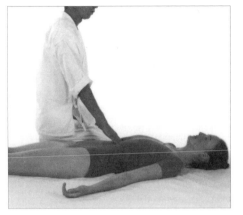

1. *Hara* diagnosis

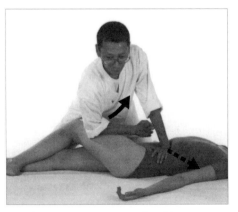

2. Hand pressure to inside of leg

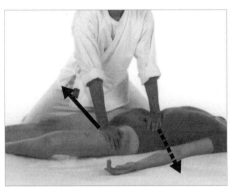

3. Ulna pressure to outside of leg

Sha: Bend the patient's right leg over the left and apply ulna pressure to the outside of the leg. Repeat twice on each of three points on the upper leg and three points on the lower leg. Bend the patient's left leg over the right and repeat the procedure on the left leg.

4. Ulna pressure to the front of the thigh (Stomach Meridian)

Posture: Straighten the patient's leg.

Ho: Place your left hand on the patient's *hara*.

Sha: Apply ulna pressure to three points on the front of both thighs. Repeat twice.

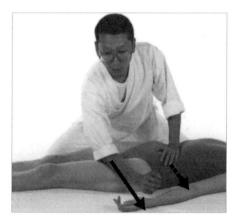

4. Ulna pressure to thigh

5. Thumb and index finger clipping pressure to the lower leg

Posture: Sit at the patient's feet, facing the patient.

Apply thumb and index finger clipping pressure to both sides of the tibia line on three points between the patient's knees and ankles. Repeat twice.

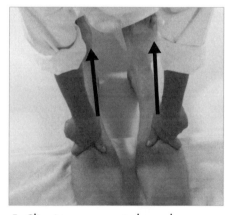

5. Clipping pressure to lower leg

6. Knee pressure to the back of the thighs

Posture: Sit alongside the patient's left leg. Bend the patient's left knee and clasp your hands around it.

A. (Kidney Meridian) Place your left knee on the back of the patient's left thigh and apply pressure by leaning backward. Repeat twice on three points. (This photo depicts the procedure for the patient's right thigh.)

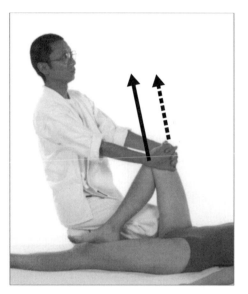

6 A. Knee pressure to back of thigh

B. (Large Intestine Meridian) The position is the same as (A), but the knee pressure is directed diagonally toward the patient's right shoulder.

Repeat A and B on the patient's right thigh.

7. Correction of the lumbar vertebrae

Ho: Place your right palm on the front of the patient's left shoulder. (This photo depicts the procedure for the patient's right side.)

Sha: Take the patient's left knee with your left hand and move the knee toward the patient's chest,

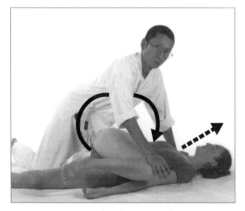

7. Correction to lumbar vertebrae

rotating it across to the patient's right side. Once only.

Repeat on the patient's right side.

8. Extension of the inside of the legs

Ho: Grasp the patient's toes with both hands and spread the legs slightly.

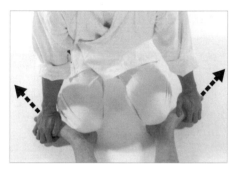

8. Extension of inside of legs

Sha: Place your knees on the patient's insteps.

9. Completion on the legs

A. Grasp the tips of the toes and shake them up and down as though to shake the patient's whole body.

B. Grasp both feet almost at the ankle with the thumb at the instep. Draw out *ki* from the toes by taking up slack and then letting go of the feet.

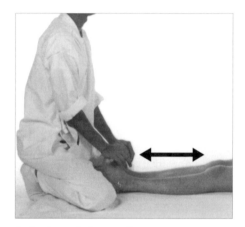

9 A. Completion on legs

10. Palm pressure to the back area

Posture: Ask the patient to sit up. Place yourself behind the patient.

Ho: Hold the patient's left shoulder with your left hand.

Sha: Apply palm pressure with your right hand to three points along the spine. Repeat twice.

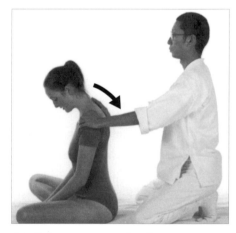

10. Palm pressure to back

11. Grasping pressure to the neck area

Posture: Raise your hips.

Ho: Place your left hand on the patient's forehead.

Sha: With the whole of the right palm, apply grasping pressure to three points on the neck. Repeat twice.

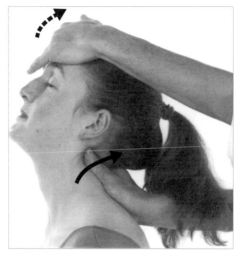

11. Grasping pressure to neck area

12. Ulna pressure to the arms

Posture: Raise your right knee and position it under the patient's armpit. Place the patient's left arm on your right thigh.

Ho: Support the patient's wrist with your left hand.

Sha: Apply right ulna pressure on several points from the top of the shoulder to the forearm.

Repeat twice.

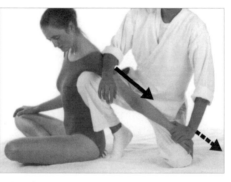

12. Ulna pressure to arms

13. Forearm extension

Ho: Place your right hand on the patient's wrist.

Sha: With your left hand, flex the patient's hand backward to stretch the underside of the forearm. Once only.

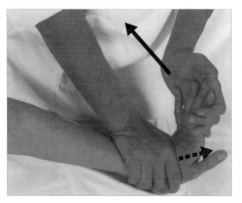

13. Forearm extension

14. Exercising the arms

Ho: Place your right hand on the patient's left shoulder blade.

Sha: With your left hand, hold the patient's elbow and rotate the patient's arm widely. Repeat three times.

15. Elbow pressure to the back area

Ho: Hold the patient's left shoulder with your left hand.

Sha: Place your right elbow between the shoulder blade and spine. Apply right elbow pressure while drawing the patient's shoulder back with your left hand. Repeat twice on four points, between the shoulder blade and spine.

Repeat steps 11–15 on the patient's right side.

16. Pressure of both knees on the hip area

Ho: Hold the patient's shoulders with your hands.

Sha: Place both knees on the patient's sacrum and apply pressure with the knees while drawing the patient's shoulders toward you.

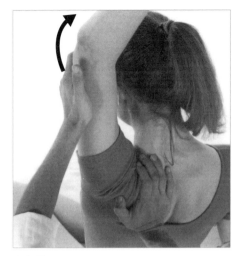

14. Exercising arms

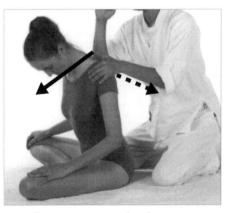

15. Elbow pressure to back

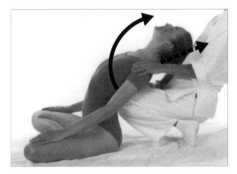

16. Knee pressure to hip area

Repeat twice on three points from the bottom up.

17. Grasping pressure using both thumbs on back area

Posture: Stand.

Place the fingers of both hands on the top of the patient's shoulder blades. Use your thumbs simultaneously between the shoulder blades in a rotating, kneading movement to draw in the skin on the patient's back.

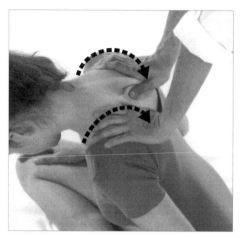

17. Grasping pressure to back area

18. Completion on sitting position

Posture: Place the outside of your left leg against the patient's back.

A. Hold the patient's elbows and rotate the arms while stretching them out. Repeat three times.

B. In the same position, hold the patient's wrists and lean your body backward, extending the patient's arms and lowering them.

C. With the palms of your hands, stimulate the flow of *ki* by brushing the back, the arms, and the back again, in that order.

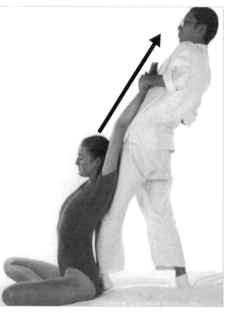

18 B. Completion

19. Hand-walking on and extending the arms

Posture: Ask the patient to lie down again, face up. Place yourself at the head of the patient.

"Walk" your whole hands down the patient's arms from the shoulders to the wrists. Then take hold of the patient's wrists and draw the arms toward you, leaning backward.

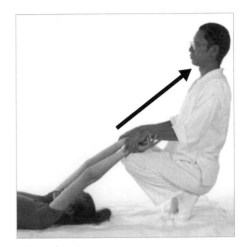

19. Extending arms

20. Fist pressure to the chest muscles

Using both hands, apply fist pressure to one point below the shoulders as if to open up the chest. Repeat twice.

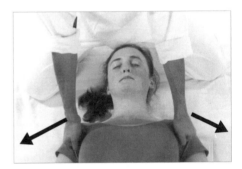

20. Fist pressure to chest

21. Four finger pressure to the back of the neck

Cup your hands with the palms facing up and apply four finger pressure to raise the neck as if to raise it with your fingers. Repeat twice on three points on the nape of the neck.

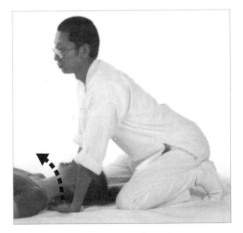

21. Pressure on back of neck

22. Grasping pressure to the neck and one-point thumb pressure to the back of the head

Ho: Bend the patient's head to the right and place your right palm on the patient's temple.

Sha: With your left hand, apply grasping pressure to the neck area. Repeat twice on three points.

Repeat on the opposite side.

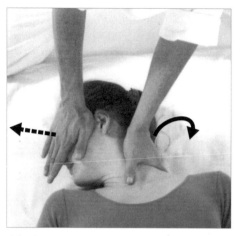

22. Grasping pressure to neck

23. Four finger pressure to the lower part of the back of the head

With the back of your hands on the floor, place four fingers on the base of the patient's head and pull the head toward you while raising and lowering the head. Repeat several times.

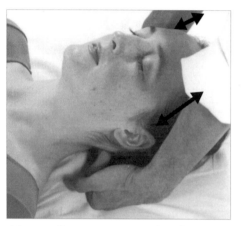

23. Four finger pressure to head

24. Finger pressure to the head and face

A. Apply pressure to the forehead with both palms. Repeat twice.

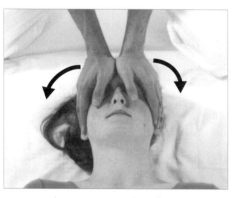

24 A. Palm pressure to head

B. Apply circular pressure with all fingers on three points on the face: the Small Intestine Meridian (the lower side of the cheekbone); the Large Intestine Meridian (the mental foramen, around the temple); the Gall Bladder Meridian (the tips of both eyebrows).

C. Apply pressure with both thumbs to the *hyakue* point (also known as *kundalini* in Indian Yogic practice), which is at the very center of the top of the head. Repeat twice.

D. Cup hands on both ears and both eyes for two or three seconds each, as if to block them.

E. Brush *ki* in the sides and top of the head from the neck. Once only.

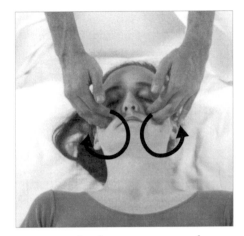

24 B. Circular finger pressure to face

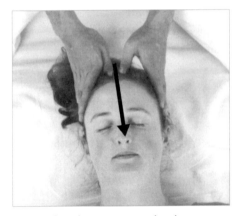

24 C. Thumb pressure to *hyakue* point

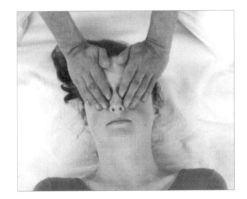

24 D. Cupping hands over eyes

25. Ulna pressure to the arms

Posture: Sit to the left of the patient with your right thigh under the patient's left arm.

Ho: Place your right hand on the patient's left wrist, taking up the slack of the skin toward the finger-tips.

Sha: With your left ulna, apply pressure to several points on the patient's arm, from the shoulder to the wrist. Repeat twice.

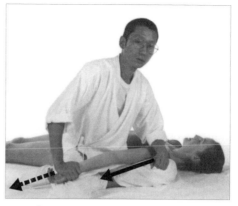

25. Ulna pressure to arms

26. Knee pressure to the upper arm

Posture: Face the patient, still sitting near the left shoulder.

Apply knee pressure to the upper arm and lean back in the same way as in step 6. Repeat twice on three points.

27. Knee pressure to the forearm

Posture: Place the patient's palms on the floor.

Ho: Place your left hand on the patient's left wrist and your right hand on the patient's upper arm.

Sha: With your left knee, apply pressure to the forearm. Repeat twice on three points.

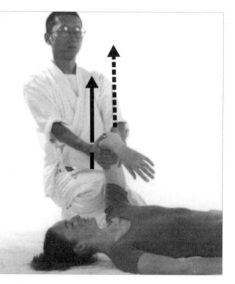

26. Knee pressure to upper arm

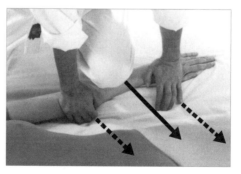

27. Knee pressure to forearm

Repeat steps 25–27 on the right arm.

28. Palm pressure to the *hara* area

Posture: Sit with your thigh placed against the right side of the patient's torso.

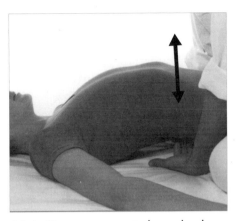

28 A. Finger pressure to lower back

A. Place your hands around the patient's waist with your fingers on the patient's lower back, pressing upward as if to raise the patient. Repeat on three points down toward the sacrum.

B. Place both palms on the lower abdomen and gradually move them in time with the patient's breath: lift the palms slightly away from the body with each inhalation and keep them still with the exhalation. When your hands are completely away from the patient's body, your *ki* remains in the *hara* area, and the patient is left with the feeling that your hands are still on his or her abdomen.

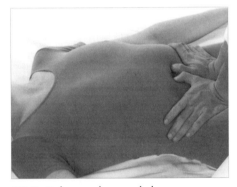

28 B. Palms on lower abdomen

This completes the basic forms of Tao shiatsu. Among these forms, shiatsu therapy on the patient lying on his or her side is usually performed as the basic treatment.

Shiatsu for Children

Shiatsu performed on children should only use the palm, the heel of the hand, the thumbs, and the fingers, which give soft pressure. The knees and elbows are not used. Shiatsu for children is technically very simple and can be performed easily, even by amateurs. It is an abbreviated basic form of Tao shiatsu.

This type of shiatsu may be practiced on sick children by professional healers, but it is more usefully practiced by the children's mother or father. Once parents learn these techniques, they are able to perform shiatsu therapy on their sick children every day. Even in clinical practice, if the patient is a child, the parent is taught these basic techniques. This is because nothing is more beneficial for children than a parent's loving hands. In fact, diseases such as asthma can actually be cured by the parent's hands.

Average people who acquire such understanding can use it not only on sick children but also on other family members. True health is heightened by physical contact with the people in one's immediate vicinity. Because environments are created by each and every person who lives within them, physical contact is fundamental to the development of an ideal, peaceful society. The power of positive change in the world does not lie in the government or other institutions but within the minds of those who fully accept the existence of other people and communities. One way of promoting this acceptance is to spread the knowledge of such basic techniques as shiatsu for children to people in general.

Lying on Side

1. Palm pressure to the left leg

With your left hand on the child's ankle, apply right palm pressure to the child's left leg. Repeat twice on several points.

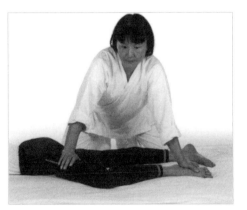

1. Palm pressure to leg

2. Clipping pressure to the foot

With your right hand on the child's left ankle, apply clipping pressure to the foot with your left hand. Repeat twice on three points.

3. Heel of the hand pressure to the right leg

With your left hand on the child's right foot, apply heel of the hand pressure to the leg with your right hand. Repeat twice on several points.

4. Thumb pressure to the bottom of the right foot

Apply thumb pressure by holding the foot between the thumb and fingers of both your hands. Repeat twice on three points.

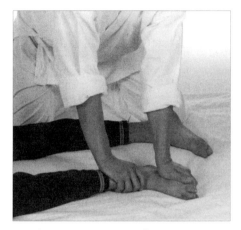

2. Clipping pressure to foot

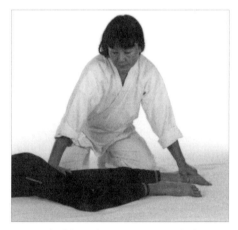

3. Heel of hand pressure to right leg

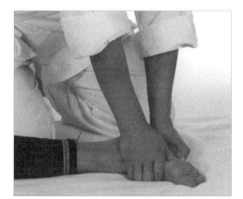

4. Thumb pressure to foot

5. Heel of the hand pressure to the side of the head

With your right hand on the back of the head, use your left hand to apply heel of the hand pressure to the side of the head. Repeat twice on three points.

6. Palm pressure to the side of the face

Keeping your right hand on the back of the head, move your left hand to the child's face and apply heel of the hand pressure. Repeat twice on three points.

7. Grasping pressure to the neck

With your left hand on the front of the child's shoulder, use your right hand to apply grasping pressure to the neck. Repeat twice on three points.

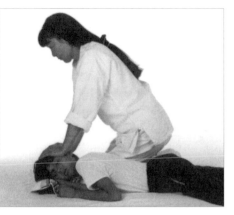

5. Heel of hand pressure to head

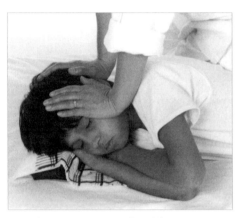

6. Palm pressure to side of face

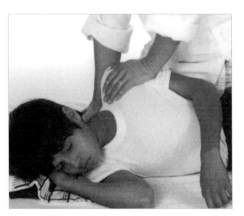

7. Grasping pressure to neck

8. Two finger pressure to the back of the shoulder

Align yourself so that your shoulders are parallel with the child's body. Place your left hand on the child's shoulder blade and apply two finger pressure to the shoulder with your right hand. Repeat twice on three points.

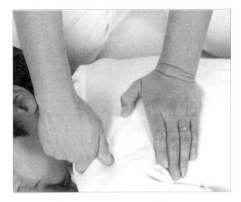

8. Two finger pressure to shoulder

9. Grasping pressure to the left arm

Posture: Straighten the child's left arm so that the back of the hand is on the floor.

Ho: Place your left hand on the child's left hand.

Sha: Apply grasping pressure to the upper arm with your right palm. Repeat twice on several points from the upper arm to the wrist.

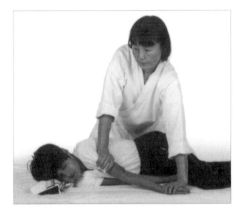

9. Grasping pressure to arm

10. Exercising the arm

Rotate the child's left arm three times.

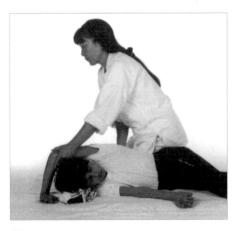

10. Exercising arm

11. Extension of the side of the body

Place your right hand on the child's elbow and your left hand on the child's lower back and move your hands in opposite directions to stretch the side of the body. Hold for several seconds.

12. Arm extension

Hold the child's arm and shoulder to your thigh and extend the arm by leaning back.

13. Thumb pressure to the back

Posture: Align yourself with the child so that the outside of your left thigh is near the child's sacral bone.

Ho: Place your left hand on the child's waist.

Sha: Apply thumb pressure to the child's back, using your fingers for support. Repeat twice on several points.

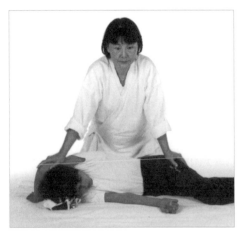

11. Extension of side of body

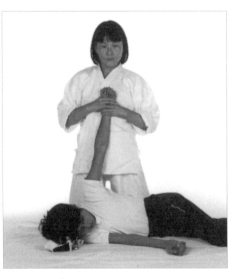

12. Extending arm

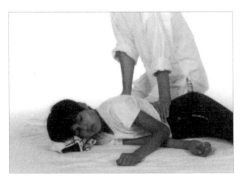

13. Thumb pressure to back

14. Fist pressure to the hip area

Posture: Place yourself perpendicular to the child.

Ho: Place your right hand on the side of the child's torso.

Sha: Apply fist pressure to the child's hip area with your left hand. Repeat twice on three points.

15. Extension of the side of the body

Place your left hand on the child's lower left thigh and your right hand on the front of the child's left shoulder. Use both hands to stretch the child's body.

Repeat steps 1–15 on the child's right side.

16. Completion

A. With your right hand, apply palm pressure to the child's back. Once on three points.

B. Stimulate the flow of *ki* by rubbing the child's entire back area gently with the palm of your hand.

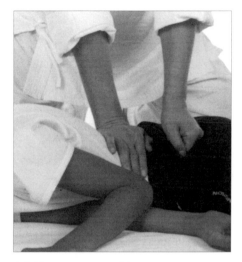

14. Fist pressure to hip area

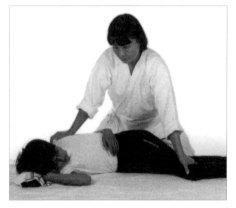

15. Extending side of body

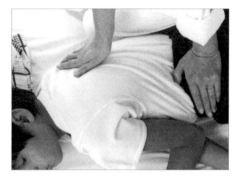

16 A. Palm pressure to back

Lying Face Down

1. Walking the hands on the back and arms

Using your whole hands, "walk" down the back and left arm.

2. Thumb pressure to the back

Place your left hand on the child's shoulder and apply thumb pressure to the left side of the child's back. Repeat twice on several points.

3. Two finger pressure to the sacral bone

Place your left hand on the child's lower back. With your right hand, apply two finger pressure to the child's sacral bone. Repeat twice on three points.

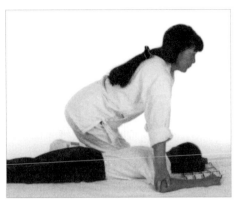

1. Walking hands on arms

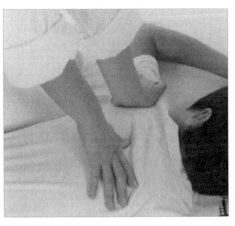

2. Thumb pressure to back

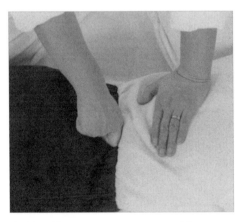

3. Two finger pressure to sacral bone

4. Two finger pressure to the hips

Place your left hand on the child's lower back. With your right hand, apply two finger pressure to the child's hips. Repeat twice on three points.

5. Heel of the hand pressure to the thighs

Place your left hand on the child's sacral bone area. With your right hand, apply heel of the hand pressure to the child's left thigh. Repeat twice on three points.

6. Palm pressure to the lower leg

Place your left hand on the child's thigh. With your right hand, apply palm pressure to the child's lower leg. Repeat twice on three points.

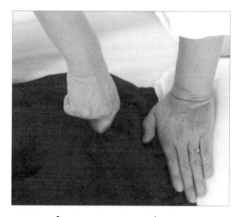

4. Two finger pressure to hips

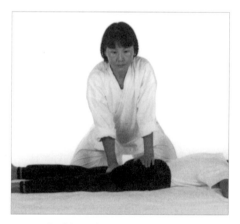

5. Heel of hand pressure to thighs

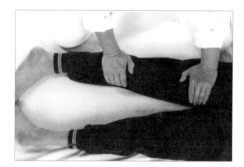

6. Palm pressure to lower leg

7. Thumb pressure to the bottom of the foot

Using both thumbs, apply pressure to the bottom of the child's foot. Repeat twice on three points.

Repeat steps 1–7 on the right side.

8. Leg extension

Grasp the child's feet with both hands. Stretch the upper thighs by bending the legs so that the heels rest on the back of the thighs.

9. Palm pressure to the leg

Place your right hand on the child's buttock and apply palm pressure to the left leg. Repeat twice on four points and then repeat on the right leg.

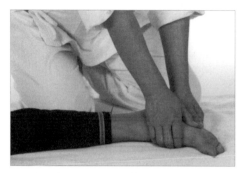

7. Thumb pressure to foot

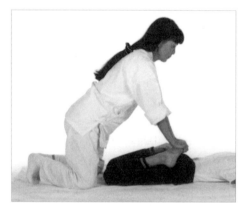

8. Leg extension

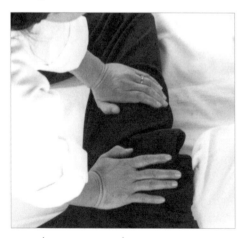

9. Palm pressure to leg

10. Completion

A. Place both palms on the child's shoulders and slide up and down. Repeat on the lower back, the hip area, and the buttocks.

B. Rub the back area gently with the palms of your hands. Repeat twice.

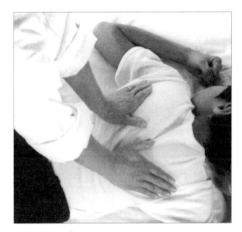

10. Completion

Lying Face Up and Sitting

1. Palm pressure to the *hara* area

Place your left hand under the child's lower back area. With your right hand, apply palm pressure from the pit of the stomach to the lower abdomen. Repeat twice on three points.

2. Heel of the hand pressure to the *hara* area

Using the heel of your right hand, apply pressure to random points in the *hara* area.

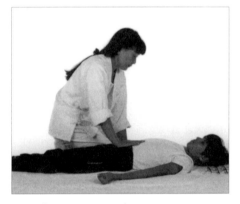

1. Palm pressure to *hara*

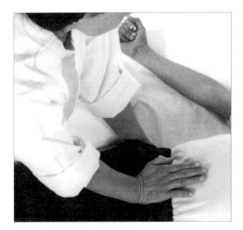

2. Hand pressure to *hara*

3. Palm pressure to the inside of the legs

Turn the child's leg out slightly, bending the knee. Place your left hand on the child's abdomen and apply right palm pressure to the inside of the leg. Repeat twice on four points on both the left and the right legs.

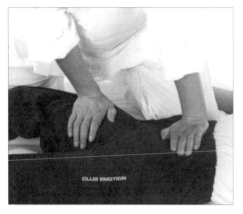

3. Palm pressure to inside of leg

4. Palm pressure to the outside of the legs

Cross the child's leg slightly over the other leg. Apply right palm pressure to the outside of the leg. Repeat twice on four points on both the left and the right leg.

5. Extension of the thighs

With your left hand on the child's lower abdomen, lift the knee with your right hand and press it toward the chest. Repeat on the other leg.

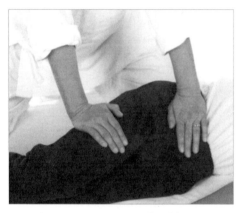

4. Palm pressure to outside of leg

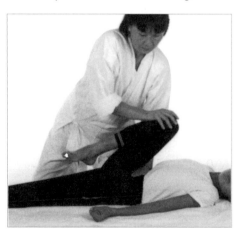

5. Extension of thigh

6. Heel of the hand pressure to the front of the thighs

With your left hand still on the abdomen, apply heel of the hand pressure to the front of the thighs. Repeat twice on three points on each leg.

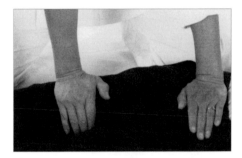

6. Heel of hand pressure to thigh

7. Two finger pressure to the lower leg

Apply two finger pressure to both sides of the shinbone. Repeat twice on three points.

8. Lowering *ki*

Sit in *seiza* and place the child's lower legs on your thighs with the bottom of the child's feet touching your abdomen. Run both palms along the child's lower legs up to the tips of the toes. This is particularly effective in lowering body temperature and should be continued for several minutes.

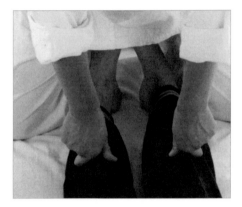

7. Two finger pressure to lower leg

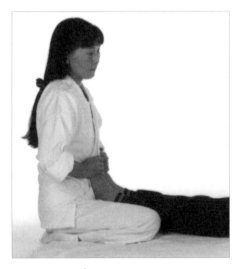

8. Lowering *ki*

9. Shaking the child's whole body

Grasp the tips of the child's toes and shake them up and down, sending vibrations throughout the child's body.

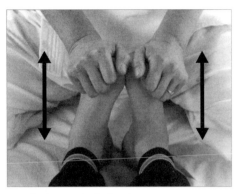

9. Shaking whole body

10. Palm pressure to the back

Ask the child to sit up. Sit behind the child. Hold the child's left shoulder with your left hand and apply palm pressure with your right hand. Repeat twice on three points.

11. Grasping pressure to the neck

Place your left hand on the child's forehead. With your right hand, apply grasping pressure to the neck. Repeat twice on three points.

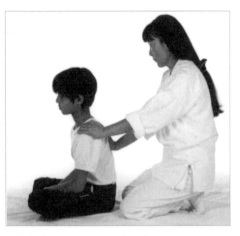

10. Palm pressure to back

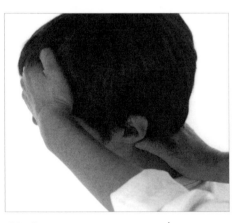

11. Grasping pressure to neck

12. Grasping pressure to the arm

Extend the child's left hand to your
thigh and hold the wrist with your
left hand. With your right hand,
apply grasping pressure to the
arm. Repeat twice on several
points.

13. Exercising the arm

Extend the child's arm and rotate
three times.

14. Thumb pressure to the back

Grasp the left shoulder with your
left hand. Apply thumb pressure to
the back with your right thumb,
using your fingers for support and
drawing the shoulder back with
your left hand. Repeat twice on
four points.

Repeat steps 12–14 on the right
side.

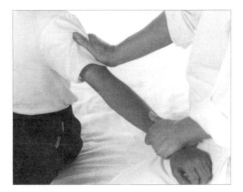

12. Grasping pressure to arm

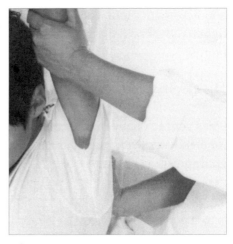

13. Exercising arm

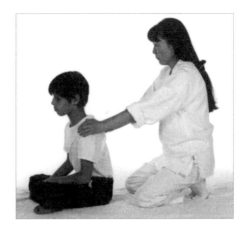

14. Thumb pressure to back

15. Extension of the arms and completion

A. Stand behind the child. Take hold of both the child's wrists and extend the arms by letting your body drop backwards. Once only.

B. Gently rub the child's back, outside of the arms, and the back again, in that order.

16. Walking the hands on the child's arms

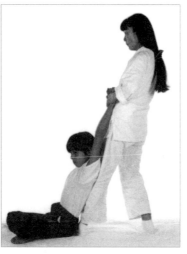

15 A. Extending arms

Ask the child to lie down again, face up. Walk your whole hands from the child's shoulders to the fingertips and back to the shoulders. Once only.

17. Moving the upper body

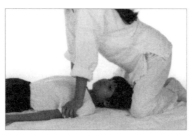

16. Walking hands on arms

Hold both the child's wrists. Draw the child's upper body upwards as if to raise his or her chin and shake gently.

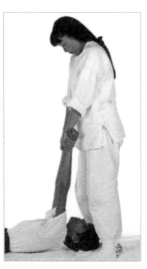

17. Moving upper body

18. Chest expansion

Place your fists on the child's shoulders and open the child's chest by pushing the shoulders downward. Once only.

19. Four finger pressure to the back of the neck

With the back of your hands on the floor, press the neck upward with your fingers as though to raise the child's chin. Repeat twice on three points.

20. Grasping pressure to the neck

Bend the child's head to the left and place your left palm on the child's temple. With your right hand, apply grasping pressure to three points on the neck, repeating twice. Repeat on the opposite side.

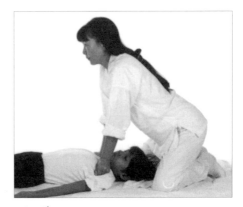

18. Chest expansion

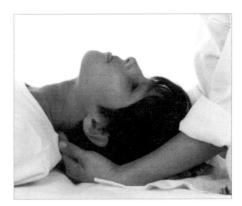

19. Four finger pressure to neck

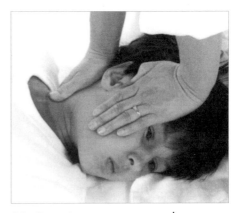

20. Grasping pressure to neck

21. Neck traction

Performed with interlaced fingers. Once only.

22. Palm pressure to the forehead

Apply pressure to the forehead with both palms. Repeat twice.

23. Four finger pressure to the face

Apply circular pressure with the four fingers around the cheek-bone, around the mouth, and on the tips of both eyebrows, in that order.

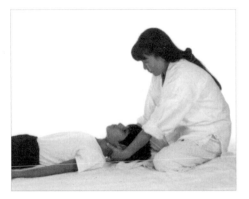

21. Neck traction

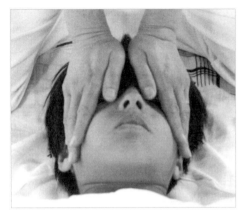

22. Palm pressure to forehead

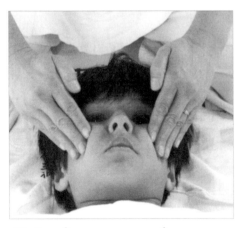

23. Four finger pressure to face

24. Thumb pressure to the top of the head

Apply pressure with both thumbs to the *hyakue* point on the top of the head. Repeat twice.

25. Touching both ears

Cup your hands over both ears, as if to block them. Hold for several seconds.

26. Touching both eyes

Cup your hands over both eyes, as if to block them. Hold for several seconds.

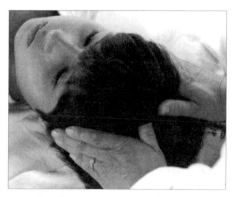

24. Thumb pressure to *hyakue* point

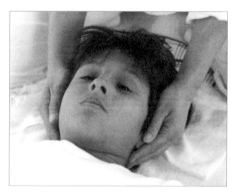

25. Touching both ears

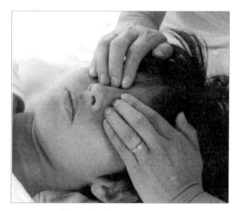

26. Touching both eyes

27. Completion on the head

Rub the sides of the child's head gently with both palms. Repeat twice.

28. Four finger pressure to the lower back area

Place your hands under the child's back, with your palms up. Press your fingers into the child's lower back as though to lift it. Repeat three times.

29. Crossing the palms over the abdomen

Cross the palms of your hands one over the other and press them on the child's abdomen for a few seconds. Remove them slowly.

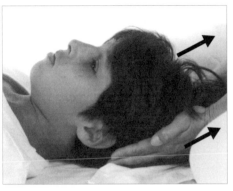

27. Completion on head

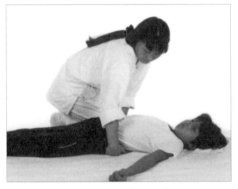

28. Finger pressure to lower back

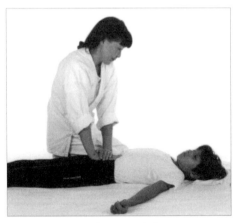

29. Crossing palms on abdomen

Chapter Three

Sho Diagnosis

What is *Sho*?

Diagnosis in Tao Shiatsu

What is generally known as "diagnosis" is the discovery of abnormalities in the body. The concept of *sho* (diagnosis of *kyo-jitsu* pattern) differs from this because it seeks to understand the patient's vital requirements. It is the healer's selection of a method of therapy according to the patient's *ki*. The differences in diagnostic methods between Oriental and Western diagnostic methods exist because of the differences between the cultures in which they are based. Western medicine distinguishes between diagnosis and treatment, and there may be cases where no method of treatment is available even after a diagnosis has been made. This is not unrelated to the fact that in Western medicine, treatment and diagnosis are carried out through complete distinction between the healer and the patient.

Western medicine has relied heavily on analysis through machinery rather than traditional methods, such as *visual, listening, dialogue*, or *touch* diagnosis (chapter 5). This has resulted in the exclusion of the subjective element from both diagnosis and treatment. Diagnosis in Oriental medicine, however, does not distinguish between the self and others and functions by sensing and responding to life. The unparalleled traditional Eastern concept of "the self and other" is reflected in Eastern medicine, in which diagnosis surpasses the subject-object perspective. Consequently, *sho* diagnosis cannot be performed within a system of medicine that replaces the human element with machinery. In the Buddhist classics, the phrase "everything is dependent on another for life" is born of a culture based on the concept that nothing exists independently as one individual body. What *sho* indicates is not an objective image of the patient's illness that reveals "something wrong," but a choice of therapy that provides the appropriate stimulation for restoring the patient's life to its original state of health.

Generally, a diagnosis that categorizes illness, such as in Western medicine, does not change as long as it is not incorrect. However, *sho* diagnosis may change even while treatment is being performed. Diagnosis in Oriental medicine adapts to treatment and does not perceive the patient objectively or statically but seeks to understand the patient dynamically. The word *sho* essentially means the "image of truth inherent in all" and is used to signify something very similar to Buddhist enlightenment. Oriental diagnosis is called *sho* because it recognizes the image of the truth of life. *Sho* diagnosis seeks to understand the direction and flow of vital *ki* energy functioning deep within the patient's mind and body. It enables the selection of appropriate herbs prescribed in Chinese herbal medicine and the selection of meridians for appropriate treatment in moxibustion, acupuncture, and shiatsu. A characteristic unique to Oriental medicine is that, through healing practices based on *sho*, the healer and the patient acquire a sympathy toward life that surpasses the subject-object antagonism.

Therefore, it may be said that the differences between Oriental and Western medicine are not in healing techniques but in attitude. When a technique of Oriental medicine is practiced through a diagnostic system that views patients analytically and manipulates their bodies, it can no longer be called Oriental medicine. On the other hand, as Masunaga emphasized in both his lectures and his writings, Western medical techniques may be valued as Oriental medicine when practiced with sympathetic understanding toward the patient.

In Oriental medicine, the patient is not simply the passive recipient of treatment, nor does his or her body undergo objective manipulation. Instead, treatment is guided by the power of healing inherent in the patient's life force. All symptoms are seen as attempts to cure illness and are a manifestation of the functions of *ki*. (For instance, diarrhea and fever may be the body's attempt to expel internal toxins.) The main aim of Oriental medicine is not to attack the symptoms directly but to heal the disorders in *ki* (the *kyo-jitsu* pattern in the meridians). Once the disturbances in *ki* have been corrected, the living body has no further need to manifest disorders and the symptoms naturally disappear.

Diagnosis in Tao shiatsu is based on the presence of the *kyo-jitsu* pattern in the meridians, which is also an indication of the patient's present physical and mental state. (For example, indications of the Gall Bladder *kyo* pattern are physical weakening of the power to digest fats and psychological decrease in the power of determination.) While conforming to the formalities of Oriental medicine, Tao shiatsu diagnosis has the definite, objective nature of modern medicine and integrates psychology and Oriental and Western medicine in order to understand the psychological significance of illness. The amount of stimulation (in other words, the dosage) is left up to the healer providing the therapy. This is because appropriate stimulation is dependent on the depth of sympathy established with the patient.

The *Kyo-Jitsu* Pattern in the Meridians

The diagnostic system that determines the *kyo-jitsu* pattern in the meridians throughout the body in Tao shiatsu is also common to Chinese medicine, acupuncture, moxibustion, and other branches of Oriental medicine. Patients who exhibit the *kyo* pattern have become ill due to a deficiency in vitality, and those who exhibit the *jitsu* pattern have become ill due to excess vitality and toxins. The *jitsu* pattern is usually prevalent in physically strong people, while the *kyo* pattern is more common in physically weaker people.[1] However, it must be understood that the *kyo-jitsu* pattern cannot be determined by comparison of numerical values, muscular strength, body weight, or other measurements. It can only be determined by comparison to universal life, in which deficiency and excess surpass contrast, are neutral and immeasurable, and can therefore only be expressed by such words as *infinite* or *nothing, empty* or *full*.

Because the *kyo-jitsu* pattern reveals the excess or deficiency of the neutral nature of universal life, in diagnosis it is also necessary to have a neutral mind that surpasses contrast and allows the healer to see the *kyo-jitsu* pattern selflessly when looking at the patient. Generally in Oriental medicine, patients who present the *kyo* pattern are treated with the *ho* method of supplementing deficient energy, and patients who present the *jitsu* pattern are treated with the *sha* method to expel the excess energy (chapter 2).

Acupuncture, moxibustion, and shiatsu all incorporate meridianal diagnosis, but there are substantial differences between the techniques. First, there is the method of *pulse diagnosis* in acupuncture and moxibustion, which is performed by placing four fingers on the radial artery. In Tao shia-

---

1. However, the "yang-*kyo* pattern," which at first glance seems to be *jitsu*, appears in predominantly *kyo*-type people. Likewise, the "yin-*jitsu* pattern," while seeming to be *kyo*, appears in predominantly *jitsu*-type people.

tsu, what is called *hara diagnosis* is performed by touch diagnosis of the abdominal area. Pulse diagnosis is a natural method that originated in China, whereas *hara* diagnosis was developed in Japan and later adopted by healers in China. What led to the development of *hara* diagnosis in Japan is the traditional Japanese focus on the *hara* (in the psychological as well as physical sense). In Japan, the *hara* (or the abdominal *tanden*) is thought to be the center of *ki* and the place where the body and mind unite. (The many phrases in Japanese such as "black *hara*," meaning slyness, and "to cut the *hara* and speak," meaning to express one's real intention, are just one indication of the cultural focus on the *hara*.) With this cultural background, practitioners of Chinese herbal medicine in Japan emphasized the abdominal area as the center of life and developed the unique form of *hara* diagnosis and therapy, generating the concept of *holistic medical healing*.

The differences between pulse diagnosis in acupuncture and *hara* diagnosis in shiatsu are that in the former, the pulse is *read* or *judged* to determine a potential cure, while the essence of the latter is the understanding of the patient's mind and spirit. Also, in acupuncture, if the pulse is normal at the time of diagnosis, treatment is deemed unnecessary in some cases. However, in shiatsu, meridianal treatment is possible in all cases. For instance, because meridianal disorders that may develop into symptoms and even illness are always present, appropriate treatment may be performed even in cases of simple fatigue. In acupuncture the object of therapy is always the symptoms; however, because shiatsu includes positive preventive medicine to enhance not only physical vitality but also the person's psychological nature, therapy may also benefit people who have no particular symptoms at the time of diagnosis. Furthermore, by performing *sho* diagnosis of the *hara* in Tao shiatsu, healers can determine disorders in the meridians before symptoms or illnesses actually appear.

Another difference between acupuncture and shiatsu is that in shiatsu the *kyo-jitsu* pattern is always diagnosed in a pair of meridians, while acupuncture sometimes carries out *kyo-jitsu* diagnosis on only one meridian. In shiatsu, one of any pair of meridians with a yin-yang relationship (for instance, the Lungs and Large Intestine, the Heart and Small Intestine) can never be *kyo* if the other is *jitsu* and vice versa. In other words, unlike in acupuncture, in shiatsu it is impossible to diagnose the Lung as *kyo* and the Large Intestine as *jitsu*. In shiatsu, *ho-sha* therapy (chapter 2) can be administered at the time of *kyo-jitsu* diagnosis, whereas acupuncture and moxibustion use the

Theory of the Five Elements of Yin and Yang, and treatment is performed not only on the meridians that present the *kyo-jitsu* pattern but also on others.

The Theory of the Five Elements of Yin and Yang

Chinese philosophy perceives the states of continuous change in nature through the mutual and antagonistic interrelationship of the five elements: wood, fire, earth, metal, and water. This is known as the Theory of the Five Elements of Yin and Yang and indicates the close relationship between Oriental medicine and Chinese philosophy. This is not simply an abstract theory based on philosophy, for its application has the possibility of achieving effective clinical results. *The Yellow Emperor's Classic of Internal Medicine* explains the relationship among the five colors, the meridians, and the five tastes, and among the five organs, voice, and musical notes. Because Chinese philosophy bases its explanation of the world of invisible *ki* on actual experience, its conclusions apply to meridianal responses in medical therapy as well. There are many examples that illustrate the close relationship between medicine and philosophy of the East. For instance, the I Ching notes that "if yin becomes extreme it eventually becomes yang"; from a meridianal perspective, when the *jitsu* pattern (yang) continues for an extended period of time, it changes into the *kyo* pattern (yin), and the reverse has also proven true in therapy. Oriental philosophy claims that "the existence of yang is based on yin," and indeed, the symptoms of the yang meridians (*jitsu*) are very easily relieved through meridianal therapy, but yin (*kyo*) symptoms cannot be felt by touch. Because yin and yang are one at their source, applying continuous steady pressure to the *kyo* and *jitsu* meridians in the *hara* area simultaneously reveals that yin and yang (*kyo* and *jitsu*) are in fact one, as are the body and mind and everything else in existence.

Figures 3.1 and 3.2 show the relationship between each of the elements, the four seasons, the tastes, the colors, and the five elements. In Figure 3.2, the solid arrows indicate the direction of the flow of *ki* energy between the elements, while the dashed arrows show the relative strengths of the meridians (an arrow leading from one element to another indicates that the first element has the power to control the second element). For instance, when practitioners of acupuncture carry out meridianal treatment using the *ho* technique on the Lung Meridian, which is wood, the Heart Meridian, which is fire and mutually related to it, becomes *jitsu*. Also, it has been clinically demonstrated that using the *sha* technique on one of a pair of meridians with the yin-yang relationship, such as the Spleen and Kidney or the Lung and Liver, causes the other to become *kyo*.

	WOOD	FIRE	EARTH	METAL	WATER
SEASON	spring	summer	Indian summer	autumn	winter
TASTE	sour	bitter	sweet	pungent	salty
COLOR	blue/green	red	yellow	white	black
MERIDIAN	liver	heart	spleen	lungs	kidney
CLIMATE	windy	hot	damp	dry	cold

Figure 3.1

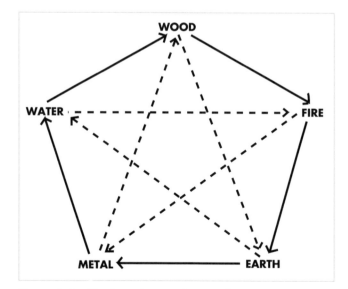

Figure 3.2   The five phases of yin and yang

Kyo-Jitsu and Personality Disorders

Fundamental to therapy in Oriental medicine is the restoration of the imbalance of the energy distorting the *kyo-jitsu* pattern to a harmonious state through which the energy of nature is circulated throughout the patient's body and mind without stagnation. Medically, *kyo* means "a state that is void of *ki* energy." Linguistically, the character for *kyo* represents something that is sunken in the middle. The character for *jitsu* indicates fullness, like a house choked with things. The *jitsu* pattern is not always positive. Just as too many possessions in a house impede movement in it and squandering money on oneself while neglecting others may lead to disaster, medically, too, extreme *jitsu* means a loss of flexibility and a toxification leading to illness. If excess energy is not used effectively, it causes stress in the mind and body. Excess mental energy may result in psychological problems such as schizophrenia, and excess physical energy can cause physical illness. For instance, chronic health problems can be caused by overconsumption of high-energy foods such as those high in protein and calories.

Kyo-jitsu patterns in the meridians may be compared to traffic conditions on roads: the *jitsu* pattern is peak-hour traffic when roads are congested with cars and progress is difficult; in the *kyo* pattern, the roads have caved in and, because it is difficult for the cars to cross, the traffic is detoured toward the *jitsu* road. Because all living bodies maintain life through desire and fulfillment of that desire, *kyo* and *jitsu* are indispensable to the vital functions of the body. For instance, when there is a lack of sustenance, the desire for food (*kyo*) is created by a drop in the blood sugar level, causing stress (*jitsu*) in the body and mind. In order to relieve this stress, the living body stimulates various functions to fulfill the desire and return to a relaxed state. The relationship between the desire or insufficiency and the action stimulated by the stress it generates also applies to the relationship between the *kyo-jitsu* pattern and the symptoms. In other words, a desire (*kyo*) creates stress (*jitsu*) and the symptoms are manifested according to this disorder. When the insufficient *ki* of *kyo* is replenished through shiatsu therapy, the patient is relieved from the stress of *jitsu* and the symptoms resolve.

This applies not only to physical illness but also to personality problems. There are many people who feel that too much love and attention spoils children. This is based on the idea that children have unlimited innate desire. Therefore these people believe that children must be scolded severely in order to learn patience. However, because these parents do not show concern for their children's true character, the children cannot improve their behavior and try to gain the parent's attention by acting spoiled. In other words, children's spoiled behavior is an expression of a desire to improve their own personality. The spoiled behavior is not the result of too much love but of insufficient true love. Children need their parents to show concern for their individual nature. In fact, because children's conscience is not yet developed, they have the logic of the Buddha Nature: the root of pre-consciousness. When parents recognize children as individuals and give them love and respect, the logic rooted in the Buddha Nature blossoms and grows. This is also an example illustrating the *kyo-jitsu* pattern; the disorder manifests itself as the child's selfish behavior (*jitsu*) which is generated by the child's desire for true love (*kyo*).

Another example is arrogance. People assume an arrogant attitude because they feel superior to others. But in fact, they are arrogant and disrespectful because they lack confidence in their own true self-worth. Their arrogant attitude is actually a desperate attempt to improve their own self-worth. If they were truly superior, they would be neither aware of nor desirous of their own superiority. Being intoxicated by a feeling of superiority means that they are comparing themselves to others and have no true peace of mind. This also illustrates *kyo* (inferiority) and *jitsu* (superiority).

Jitsu, therefore, is always generated in order to fulfill the desire of *kyo*. *Kyo-jitsu* patterns are indispensable to life because when innate desires are excluded from the living body, it becomes impossible to carry out the functions necessary to maintain life. In other words, it is because the *kyo-jitsu* pattern is generated that life functions are possible. Humans, other animals, insects, and all other living things perform life functions through the constant generation of *kyo-jitsu* patterns. Masunaga uses the example of the single-celled amoebae, which carry out necessary movements and food absorption through the functions of *solution* and *gelation*.

Masunaga writes: "When amoebae move, there is gelation (*jitsu*) at one extreme end of their original body form, which is usually in a state of solution. The process of gelation generates pseudopodium at the front end of the body form, which the organism uses as a foothold to move 'forward.' When the gelation has completed its function, the body form reverts to solution once again and the amoeba advances."[2] See Figure 3.3.

The amoeba performs its life functions through the action of solution and gelation (the *kyo-jitsu* pattern) of its cell. What causes this action is the *fluid-*

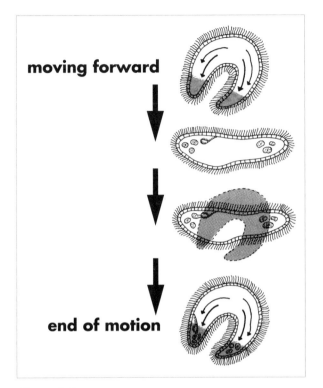

Figure 3.3

ity of its original form. As segmentation generates more cells, the original form permeates through the wall of each cell and there is a continuous exchange between cells.[3] Masunaga pursues the concept of cell generation in terms of meridians and proposes a relationship between each meridian and the *endoderm*, the *mesoderm*, and the *ectoderm*, through which the first step of segmentation from the simple cell takes place. He suggests that the Heart and Small Intestine Meridians and the Kidney and Bladder Meridians gener-

---

2. Shizuto Masunaga, *Keiraku to Shiatsu* [in Japanese] (Yokosuka: Idon Nihonsha, 1983).

3. Masunaga equates this fluidity to the meridians and maintains that the meridians are divided into the twelve-line system in much the same way as segmentation. Obviously, unlike multicellular organisms, the simple-celled ones can only be defined in terms of solution and gelation and not by the twelve-meridian system.

ate from the endoderm, which carries out the main functions of the cell. The Liver and Gall Bladder Meridians and the Spleen and Stomach Meridians generate from the mesoderm, which is responsible for the muscles and so on (see chapter 4). The Lung and Large Intestine Meridians and the Pericardium and Triple Heater Meridians generate from the ectoderm, which carries out conductivity on the epidermis.

The *Kyo-Jitsu* Pattern as the Source of Illness

Change is the essence of nature, and solution and gelation in the amoeba illustrate the changes of the *kyo-jitsu* pattern through which the indispensable vital functions are performed. However, like the solution and gelation of the amoeba, functions in the living body must be reversed after they are completed. It follows, then, that there is never a time when a *kyo-jitsu* disorder is not present, nor is there ever a state of complete fulfillment. Even the wizards and sages idealized in Oriental philosophy were not in a complete state of fulfillment. They were, however, able to harmonize with the currents of life and therefore with its relentless changes and disorders.

Illness results from the fixation of a disorder, which means that the body's flexibility—its ability to return to the original state of vitality—is lost. In other words, when a disorder loses the ability to change, the living body loses the ability to perform healthy, vital functions. Then, when the body tries to change the fixed disorder, the various symptoms of illness appear and create an opportunity for overall change. Oriental medicine does not directly attack symptoms because symptoms are seen as a part of a self-healing process through the natural changes of the body. In attempting to heal illness by stimulating changes in the body, the therapeutic direction of Oriental medicine is in complete harmony with the essential cause of the symptoms.

During therapy in Oriental medicine, before healing takes place, severe symptoms may develop, which at first glance appear to be illness. This is actually a favorable response to treatment, called the *Menken Response* (chapter 5). The severe symptoms are a reaction to the heightening of the vital force, which is able to heal the illness brought on by the symptoms. Because the essence of life lies in the normal state of change, and complete fixation means death, the source of illness is not the state where there is a disorder but the state where a disorder becomes fixed.

This ideology also explains why young people favor change: it is an expression of heightened vitality. Conversely, fixating on one thing or another and persisting in one's own feelings are both signs of mental aging. Therefore, perennial youth means acceptance of change and anticipation of challenge in all that is new. When elderly people do not maintain a heightened consciousness, they adopt a negative attitude toward others and the world and direct their attention only to themselves. In such cases, instead of mental maturity there is a loss of wisdom and virtue. Depression and isolation, by no means limited to the elderly, are also the result of overconcentration on the self. The Western psychologist Alfred Adler faces his patients suffering from depression by saying, "If you follow my instructions you will be cured in two weeks: it is beneficial for you to think about making other people happy. People who have no interest in others not only disregard human suffering but are also a cause of others' problems, and all human failure is born from among such people."[4] This approach to medical therapy indicates that the sorrows and suffering of humanity are a result of the negative thoughts revealed in the words and actions of people.

The essence of life is adaptability and change, and the opposite of this is illness, caused by the fixation of a disorder. The disorder that causes the fixation can also foster negative feelings such as anger and hate or disharmony and unfulfillment. Overattachment to work, overconsumption of unnatural foods (such as white sugar, bread made from white flour, refined rice, chemical preservatives or additives), and irregular lifestyles all result in fixation of disorders. The impulsive, emotional mind may result in fixation of the *kyo-jitsu* disorder because attachment halts the mind and causes *ki* to stagnate. The fixation of a disorder weakens vital adaptation and change and distorts the circulation of *ki*. Illness occurs when the *kyo-jitsu* disorder settles in and limits potential flow and change. The aggressive reaction of animals when humans attempt to capture them is a symptomatic vital response to the hindrance of the natural functions of the mind and body. The animal's reaction is an attempt to reactivate its vital circulation of energy.

On the other hand, it may also be said that dying of an illness is the extreme result of the exhaustion of *ki* through *excessive* response. Symptoms are one type of mental and physical energetic response. Psychiatric patients

---

4. Alfred Adler, *Understanding of Human Nature* (New York: Greenberg, 1927).

violently enrage their subconscious by trying to emerge from a state of mental fixation caused by feelings of fear toward other people and the outside world. It is said that the onset of neurosis after middle age is caused by the emergence of one part of the ego that has not been previously recognized. In such cases, the fixated conscious receives a jolt from the subconscious, which seeks change because the ego has become too deeply ingrained in society and the outside world. We generally form an attachment to our symptoms and attack them in order to improve them. Attacking the symptoms directly is the medical ideology of the West, but there are also many practitioners of acupuncture and shiatsu who perform this type of stimulating (*sha*) therapy.

Jitsu symptoms are caused by a concentration of *ki*. Stimulating the area may be effective temporarily, but, because *ki* will once again accumulate in the same place, it has no long-term benefit and there is always the possibility that the symptoms will reappear more severely than before. Superficial symptoms such as stiffness and pain often cause *jitsu* patterns in the meridians. When this pattern becomes chronic, it changes to *kyo* pain and stiffness, causing discomfort deep within the body. *Jitsu* symptoms can be resolved easily by shiatsu pressure to the *kyo* meridians that initially generated the *jitsu* pattern. Therefore, in treating the *jitsu* symptoms manifesting on the surface of the body, the healer must not lose the perspective of the whole body and must not overlook the fact that *kyo* (yin) lies behind the *jitsu* symptoms (yang). *Kyo* is holistic and because it always exists in the background and does not manifest on the surface, it is difficult to recognize.

The relationship between *kyo* and *jitsu* is directly applicable to the relationship between life (*ki*) and matter (the body). Life cannot be seen or touched, but matter is tangible and visible. The force behind the movement of physical structures is none other than the holistic vitality that surpasses contrast and differentiation. *Ki* is another name for life, and meridians play the role of mediators between the physical structures of the body and the vital force. This is because the *ki* that flows through the meridians stimulates physical movement and generates vital functions. Meridians exist as the closest connection between life and the body, and Tao shiatsu therapy heals disorders generated by the *kyo-jitsu* pattern through the direct touch of the healer's hand on the patient's body.

Perceiving *Sho*

The state of consciousness necessary for carrying out *sho* diagnosis on the meridians is dependent on a diagnostic perspective and a mental state at one of the following four depths:

1. *Kyo* diagnosis through the use of the hand in "touch diagnosis" of the *hara* area.

2. *Kyo* diagnosis through visual observation without actually touching the patient's body.

3. Diagnosis of the true source of illness as the part of the body where a *kyo* stiffness exists deep in a *kyo* meridian.

4. Recognition of the deepest level of *kyo tsubo*.

In order to arrive at some understanding of the common aspects of the various techniques of *sho* diagnosis, one must always keep the meaning of the word *kyo* in mind. *Kyo* is the world of emptiness that surpasses contrast and the background of the visible or "yang." Emptiness cannot be understood consciously and it does not mean that nothing exists. It signifies the world of the *whole*, which surpasses contrast and is absolutely free of fixation. Although the *whole* may be easily expressed in words, it is in fact more difficult to perceive as an actual sensation. The *whole* has often been described in terms of its antonym, the *part*. This is because the *part* can be acknowledged consciously, but what supports it and cannot be as easily conceptualized is the *whole*. The *part* may be a cell existing within the body (the whole), which in turn exists within an even greater *whole*: nature. In other words, because the idea of contrast cannot be surpassed, the general conscious understanding of the *whole* is *one big part*. One cannot understand the true meaning of the whole without direct experience of the Eastern view of life that "the whole is equal to the part and the part is equal to the whole." (In Buddhist terms, "all in one; one in all.") Buddhism has long understood such secrets of the holistic nature of life and views everything in terms of vibrations. Buddhist expressions such as "the oneness of the spirit and matter" signify that rough energy vibrations are matter and subtle vibrations are spirit. These are not simply philosophical phrases but direct expressions of the real form of enlightened existence attainable through discipline.

Physics proposes that energy (matter seen in a fixed state) is something that is manifested in *form* and is maintained through the constant circulation of subatomic particles. As such, it is appropriate to say that everything is made up of energy and life and what people see as fixed existence is the web of illusion of their own conscious self. Vitality is the energy in motion throughout the whole body. It has the property of *transience*, which means that it never stagnates. In shiatsu therapy, when diagnosing *kyo*, the healer does not simply look at the body as a physical structure, but empathizes with the patient's vitality (*ki*), which is the foundation of the living body. This empathy is not offered only at the time of diagnosis, for the healer who does not continue the feeling of empathy toward the patient throughout therapy cannot perform true shiatsu. Maintaining sympathy with the patient is not an easy task. However, as Tao shiatsu continues, it becomes possible to maintain a mental state of selflessness with the sole intention of empathizing with the patient's vitality. While continuing to sense the patient's vitality, the healer eventually becomes able to sense the universal life that surpasses the contrast between the self and the other, dwelling within the patient's mind. At such times the boundaries of the healer's own self broaden, and as the discipline of empathy with life advances, the healer's mental state clarifies to reflect *kyo* as clearly as an unfogged mirror reflects an object.

Sho diagnosis is not a practice in which the healer actively probes the patient's body, nor is it the search for a weak part of the body. The healer is always passive, does not pass judgment on the patient, and listens to the appeal of life with honest empathy and humility. When the healer does so, the patient develops unconscious faith in the healer and the true and fundamental direction of the purpose of therapy (the *kyo* disorder) clearly reveals itself. The absence of judgment toward others must also prevail during counseling and in everyday human relations, for *kyo* does not reveal itself to those who judge or criticize. Healers who diagnose the patient's *hara* area through physical probing tend to be overly stubborn, persistent, and locked up in their own egos. People trust and want to confide in those who listen sincerely to what is being said. Because *kyo* is patients' true reason for seeking therapy and may become their weakest point, they will not reveal *kyo* unless they sense the healer will protect it, empathize with it, and provide the energy to restore it. This is because the damage incurred when *kyo* is approached forcefully is severe enough to disturb the patient's vitality and impede physical recovery. Conversely, however, when the appropriate healer comes in contact with *kyo*, he or she may restore it from its core, enable patients to heal themselves naturally, and make it unnecessary for them to reveal symptoms and character deficiencies existing on the surface.

In such terms, the concept of diagnosing *kyo* may seem almost impossible to understand. However, *sho* diagnosis, which reveals *kyo* to the healer, is always possible through the practice of Tao shiatsu. The mind performing *sho* diagnosis is selfless and sympathetic toward the life of the patient, and its state of consciousness differs from the one based on self-interest that is pervasive in general society. At present, among those who are already involved in shiatsu therapy, some people are under the misconception that *sho* diagnosis may be performed "by applying pressure on the *hara*: what is *soft* is *kyo* and what is *hard* is *jitsu*." However, diagnosis of the *kyo-jitsu* pattern is based on levels of vitality that surpass the contrast of *soft* and *hard*.

First of all, judgment of *softness* or *hardness* is based directly on the healer's sense of touch and excludes the patient's sensations. Touch diagnosis (chapter 5) in shiatsu must always include reading the vital responses to pressure and actually feeling the patient's vital sensations as one's own. In other words, *sho* diagnosis reads the response to pressure through sympathizing with life and surpassing the distinction between the self and others, not by relying on the healer's sense of touch. Therefore, there is never any margin for judgment of the *hara* area as *soft* or *hard* by touch. *Sho* is more dignified than simple speculations on what "may be *kyo*," and it does not differ according to the diagnosing practitioner. Therefore, to those healers who truly understand *sho* diagnosis, *kyo* appears as clearly as a material object in front of their eyes. (Incorrect diagnosis is of course possible. I myself misdiagnose about one in twenty patients. This is often due to preconceptions such as expecting a patient who exhibits Lung Meridian *kyo* one week to have the same pattern the following week. Also, the healer's concentration may weaken when the healer diagnoses a number of patients in succession.)

When a healer has honest empathy with the life force of others and continues to perform meridianal therapy, eventually the patient's *kyo* will be revealed naturally, as though the healer had shed a blurring film from the eyes. *Sho* may only be attained by the healer who selflessly continues to empathize

with the patient's life. This is because empathy toward each individual corresponds to sympathy with universal life, through which the healer is then
truly able to comprehend the totality of the patient's mind and body. Empathy and awareness that actively continue to heighten the perception of *sho*
enable the healer to understand the truth of life directly: the *part* is equal to
the *whole.*

Techniques of Meridianal Diagnosis

Kyo Diagnosis

A healer begins to understand *sho* diagnosis through enhanced receptivity to
the patient's *ki.* By gaining experience in meridianal therapy, the healer can
ultimately recognize the patient's meridian that connects to the *kyo* (emptiness) of nature. From one point of view, the various methods of meridianal
diagnosis explained here are means of projecting *kyo* to the healer. From another, they are also methods that confirm whether a diagnosis is correct. The
response that appears in the *kyo* and *jitsu* meridians does not appear in any
other meridian. *Kyo* is the source of all illness, and in order to diagnose *jitsu*
it is first of all necessary to come in contact with *kyo*. *Kyo* diagnosis is carried
out through touch by placing the four fingers on the meridians in the *hara*,
revealing the following characteristic responses:

1. The *kyo* meridians are those where the patient most requires *ki.*

2. When pressure is applied to the *kyo* meridians, the whole body relaxes.

3. When pressure is applied to the *kyo* meridians in the *hara* area, the symptoms improve or disappear.

4. When pressure is applied to the *kyo* meridians in the *hara* area, the
   healer's *ki* spreads throughout the patient's body.

Hara Kyo:*Where the Patient Most Requires *Ki. *Jitsu* meridians are characteristically tense and hard, while *kyo* meridians are weak and without resistance. However, as this is not always the case, these characteristics cannot be used as standard diagnostic criteria. Because the *kyo* meridians are a manifestation of the deficiency of *ki*, their weakness and lack of resistance may be felt through touch when pressure is applied. However, correct *sho* cannot be perceived if the sense of touch is the basis for diagnosis. This is because, even though resistance and relative hardness are discerned through the healer's sense of touch, initially *sho* diagnosis is based on the patient's response to pressure. In fact, when pressure is applied to *kyo* meridians, they often recede. But not all *kyo* meridians are limited to such objective characteristics. There are some that are *hard* on the surface (like *jitsu*) and *soft* underneath, and some that appear to be hard when pressed. *Kyo* meridians in the limbs sometimes soften and reveal their true nature in the *hara* for the first time long after treatment has begun.

The reasons not to rely on the sense of touch for diagnosis have less to do with potential errors in diagnostic conclusions than with the disruption caused by the healer's ability to discern *softness* or *hardness.* To perform truly accurate *sho* diagnosis, the healer must surpass his or her own sense of touch and actually feel the sensations of the patient's life. Recognizing *kyo* signifies sympathetic recognition of the meridians that need to be treated with *ki.* In other words, *kyo* is an understanding of which meridians are demanding shiatsu through the patient's subconscious. Therefore, diagnostic conclusions of *hardness* or *softness* by simple application of pressure cannot have the same effect as sympathy with the patient, and this is not an appropriate method of *sho* diagnosis because it excludes consideration of the patient's vital sensations.

To perform *sho* diagnosis, the healer must first of all surpass his or her own self and earnestly sympathize with the patient's response to pressure. For instance, in meridianal diagnosis, if the mind is pure and in sympathy with the patient, pressing the Lung Meridian facilitates inhalation, and pressing the Triple Heater Meridian stimulates feelings of well-being. According to such responses to pressure, the healer becomes able to easily distinguish and understand the different response of each meridian. Meridians are perceived through this response to pressure and not through an understanding of their position in the physical body. Furthermore, it is important to remember that the body changes depending on the individual and his or her circumstances, and may even change from one day to the next.

Touch diagnosis recognizes the differences in response to pressure generated by changes in the patient's *ki*. For instance, in touch diagnosis of the Large Intestine Meridian in the *hara* area, the healer knows he or she is indeed touching the Large Intestine Meridian not because the pressure is being applied to the right place but because the pressure stimulates a response in the Large Intestine Meridian throughout the body. Therefore the meridians in the *hara* shown in meridianal diagrams are not an indication of where the meridians are actually positioned but of the part of the body where a response may appear. Furthermore, by applying pressure to one part of the body, the healer may diagnose the state of the meridians in the whole body. Touch diagnosis of the meridians in the *hara* is a method through which the healer may form direct contact with the patient's vital sensations. The gateway to *kyo-jitsu* diagnosis is the healer's disregard for the sense of touch in his or her own fingers and selfless attempt to read the patient's response to pressure. Diagnosis or treatment must never be performed by a hand skilled only in technique, for at the time of diagnosis the only thing the healer can truly rely on is his or her sympathy with the patient's life. Enriching and nourishing the healer's sense of sympathy leads the healer to understand which meridians lack vitality and most require *ki*.

Relaxing the Whole Body. Pressing the *kyo* meridians with sympathetic hands stimulates a deep relaxed state throughout the patient's body. This is a unique life sensation recognized by sensing the meridians responsible for the patient's *kyo* pattern, and it does not occur when the meridians pressed are not *kyo*. The relaxed sensation is the source of *kyo* felt as a pervasive emptiness and is in some ways the most characteristic aim of diagnosis.

However, when the meridians in the *hara* are indicated on the surface (see diagrams of meridians), even if they are *kyo*, simple application of pressure does not stimulate the relaxation response. In such cases, if the meridians in the limbs are treated first, pressing the *kyo* in the *hara* clearly stimulates the relaxation response. This happens because *kyo* is a point of weakness and the skin and superficial muscles function defensively in order to shield it. If the patient is relatively healthy, diagnosis of the *hara* area through simple touch may stimulate something similar to the relaxation response, because the body does not react defensively. In such cases, the true relaxation response appears clearly if the meridians in the limbs are treated first and then the defense response is relieved by pressing the *kyo* in the *hara*.

The meridians in the *hara* area are not only those that appear in these diagrams but all the meridians, including those running vertically and horizontally. For instance, if touch diagnosis of the *hara* area is only intended to reach the depth of the Lung Meridian, which runs both vertically and horizontally, it does not reach the depth of the Stomach Meridian. Therefore, the relaxation response resulting from touch diagnosis of the *hara* to determine the *kyo-jitsu* pattern is in this case due to the Lung Meridian and not the Stomach Meridian. This is an indication that correct *sho* diagnosis cannot be carried out by the healer who seeks to confirm through the sense of touch which meridian he or she is diagnosing. Meridians run much more deeply than the skin. The same meridian differs in depth in different parts of the body, and each meridian's depth is different from the rest. The meridians in the *hara* are more deeply positioned than the others. This is not apparent in diagrams, where the meridians all seem to be stacked up together in some places because they are only shown in two dimensions.

Taking all this into consideration, it can be said that the relaxation response, which is the aim of meridianal diagnosis in the *hara*, is not at all an easy one to attain. This is first because even if one presses the *kyo* in the *hara*, the relaxation response may not occur. Second, even if the response appears, unless the healer has heightened receptivity, he or she cannot determine the most effective meridian for touch diagnosis. However, producing the relaxation response is not totally impossible. First of all, the healer must select several meridians in the *hara* where he or she senses the patient's desire for shiatsu pressure. Among these meridians, the healer should then select the ones judged most likely to induce a relaxed state throughout the body by applying pressure to the *tsubo* at the extremities of the body, such as those in the wrist or the foot. As the healer applies pressure, it will become apparent which meridians induce a state of relaxation throughout the body: these are the *kyo* meridians.

One reason why applying pressure to the *tsubo* in the wrists or the feet facilitates accurate diagnosis is that these *tsubo* are fixed whereas meridians shift and change constantly. The healer should be aware that even though there is less possibility of error when using these *tsubo* compared to those in other parts of the body, mistakes are nonetheless possible when diagnosing the sub-meridians and those that run horizontally throughout the body. However, when a meridianal response does not occur even after pressing the *kyo* in the *hara*, applying pressure to the *tsubo* in the extremities of the body can induce a response. In other words, a relaxed response can always be produced by pressing the *tsubo* in either the hands or the feet.

When judging the relaxed response to pressure on the wrists or feet, it is advisable to ask the patient which points produce the most relaxed state throughout the body. However, there are many people whose primal sense is dulled and who cannot easily reply to this question. In such cases the healer should press two meridians alternately and determine *kyo* through elimination by asking which of the two is most relaxing. For example, when comparing the Lung and Large Intestine Meridian, if the patient replies that pressing the Lung Meridian is more relaxing, eliminate the Large Intestine Meridian and take the Lung Meridian to be *kyo*.

Furthermore, *softness* or *hardness* of *jitsu* resulting from pressure applied to the *kyo* meridians cannot definitely reveal whether the healer's diagnosis of the *kyo-jitsu* pattern is correct. This is because even if the pattern is not true *kyo*, there are *kyo*-type meridians that can soften *jitsu*. A true *kyo* meridian is selected on the basis that it will always generate the most relaxed state throughout the body. Therefore, one indication that a meridian is definitely *kyo* is that it produces a relaxed response throughout the body when pressure is applied to the *tsubo* in the wrists and feet.

Jitsu Symptoms Disappear and Kyo Symptoms Improve. In cases where the symptoms are pain or stiffness, if they are *jitsu*, they may be easily removed by treating the corresponding *kyo*. However, if the symptoms are *kyo*, it is not quite as simple. One interesting phenomenon of *kyo* and *jitsu* can be seen in a contusion incurred suddenly. Pressing the *kyo* in the *hara* area and applying relatively strong pressure to the *kyo* meridians in the legs relieves the pain, but as soon as the application of pressure ceases, the pain returns. Furthermore, all symptoms may disappear when the healer applies strong, continuous pressure to several points on the meridians in the limbs (the legs in particular). Treatment of the leg or arm opposite to the painful side also has an effective result on *jitsu* symptoms.

When using these practices in diagnosis, healers should perform touch diagnosis and look for the parts of the body that have taken on the symptoms of pain or stiffness. The *jitsu* symptoms can be relatively easily relieved by pressing the *kyo* meridians in the legs or the *hara* area, which also makes it possible to determine the *kyo* meridians.[5] However, symptoms caused by disorders in *ki*, even though they are subtle and promptly revealed through relaxation, may not be as easily relieved by pressure on the *hara* area or legs.

Sensing the Spread of *Ki* throughout the Body. When the receptivity of the healer's *ki* is heightened, the healer can feel the patient's *ki* through his or her response to the given pressure. It is possible to diagnose the true source of *kyo* once this standard is reached. This is because when the healer who is able to sense *ki* performs touch diagnosis on the meridians in the patient's *hara* area, he or she is able to understand the difference in response to pressure as the difference in the scope of the "spreading *ki*" (generated by applying pressure to the meridians in the *hara* area). In other words, pressure to the meridians in the *hara* area is extended throughout the body by the *kyo* meridians, therefore spreading *ki*. (Applying pressure to meridians that are not *kyo* does not spread *ki* throughout the whole body.)

There is no other means of explaining the phenomenon of the spreading of *ki*, and there is no method for students to acquire this experience other than enhancing their own receptivity toward *ki* through self-discipline.

Kyo Diagnostic Method

To diagnose *kyo*, follow these three steps.

1. *Choosing Four Meridians through Touch Diagnosis.* Using the points of diagnosis on the *hara* region shown in chapter 4 for the fourteen meridians, the healer should select as many as four that may be *kyo*. The healer's thoughts in determining which meridians to choose must always be, "when the patient is pressed here, he or she relaxes, when pressed here, he or she will feel good," and so on, always making the patient's sensations (the response to pressure) the subject. The healer must never depend on the relative hardness sensed through touch.

2. *Carrying Out the O-Ring Test Based on the Four Meridians.* Locate the selected four meridians in the *hara* area and perform the O-Ring Test

---

5. Confirming to patients that neck and shoulder stiffness can be relieved by shiatsu to the *hara* is advantageous because it helps them to understand the efficiency of meridianal therapy.

(described below) by using the pieces of paper with the names of the four meridians written on them. Select the meridians that allow the ring to open most easily.

3. *Selecting the True Kyo Meridians.* Among the pairs of meridians written on the pieces of paper, select the ones that have a true *kyo* nature by pressing the main meridians on the wrist or the sub-meridians on the bottom of the foot. The *kyo* meridians are the ones that respond by relaxing the whole body. To support the diagnostic decision, the healer may also ask the patient to touch the *kyo* area with the fingertips of his or her left hand and perform the O-Ring Test. The *kyo* meridians are those that, when touched by the patient, allow the O-Ring to open easily.

The O-Ring Test. Masayasu Katsuta describes the O-Ring Test as follows (see Figure 3.4):

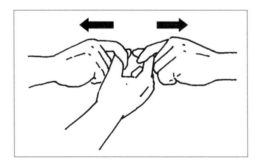

Figure 3.4

The O-Ring Test, more precisely known as the "Bi-digital O-Ring Test," is a method of diagnosis that Professor Yoshiaki Omura, a leading scholar in the research of cardiac disease, developed from kinetology (a functional study of the practical use of movement developed by American chiropractor George Guthart). It is a convenient method of diagnosis that can promptly determine virulence, reveal abnormalities in the body's organs without the use of complex diagnostic tools, and determine whether a drug is effective.

The patient and the analyst face each other and the patient makes an O shape with the right hand (or the hand most used) by touching the tip of the thumb to the tip of the index finger. The analyst inserts both index fingers through the circle, making two circles through the patient's O-Ring by touching the tips of the thumbs with the tips of the index fingers. The analyst then tries to open the patient's ring by pulling it apart with the two rings made by his or her own fingers, as shown in figure [3.4]. The patient tries to resist this by holding the ring closed tightly. At this point, the analyst determines the amount of strength in the patient's fingers according to the degree of strength required to open the O-Ring.

Patients must first of all take off rings, metal belts, necklaces, watches, and any other metallic garment or object they might be wearing. They may be sitting, standing, or lying down. They should let their feet open slightly and must not allow either arm to touch the side of their own body. The analyst places medicine (or drink, food, etc.) in the patient's left hand and performs the O-Ring test on the right hand. If the food product or medicine in the left hand is toxic, the O-Ring will open easily. If it is an inappropriate medicine, food, or drink, the strength in the patient's fingers weakens in response.[6]

For instance, when a cigarette or a sweet made from white sugar is placed in the patient's left hand for the O-Ring Test, the ring can be opened very easily. The results are the same when the test is repeated with a bottle of whiskey or other alcoholic beverage in the patient's left hand.[7] The O-Ring Test is not only convenient for diagnosis but also for determining appropriate dosage of medication or stimulation to be prescribed. The important thing to consider in carrying out this test is that both the analyst and the patient must be in a passive state of mind. When the O-Ring Test is performed on patients who have a strong will, they may be determined not to allow the ring to open regardless of how strong the toxin in the left hand may be, and the ring does not open. Conversely, if the analyst is of strong will and determined to succeed,

---

6. Masayasu Katsuta, *Ki o Meguru Boken* [in Japanese] (Tokyo: Hajusha, 1989).
7. Professor Katsuta explains that people who like whiskey and water (a very popular drink in Japan) do not consider this drink to be detrimental to their health, and for these people the experiment has different results.

he or she can make any ring open. Although such people do not negate the real value of the O-Ring Test as an effective method of diagnosis, unless both the analyst and the patient become passive during the test, the results may not be conclusive.

Professor Katsuta goes on to explain that in *qigong*, anesthesia using the spot in the middle of the forehead known as the third eye (see Figure 3.5) can make patients fall asleep, and that tests of Chinese herbal medicine carried out on this spot are even more effective than on the palm of the hand. He also states that if a piece of paper on which the name of a drug is written is applied to the middle of the forehead, the results are as effective as when applying the drug itself. Following these suggestions, the O-Ring Test has also been performed by placing a piece of paper with the names of the meridians on the patient's forehead. That is, the names of the pairs of meridians—Lung and Large Intestine, the Governor and Conception Vessels, and so on—are written on seven different pieces of paper and the papers are placed one at a time on the patient's forehead. The meridians that allow the O-Ring to open most easily are *kyo*.

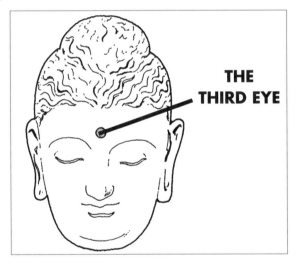

Figure 3.5

Jitsu **Diagnostic Method**

Basic meridianal treatment is sufficient to resolve *kyo* stiffness; but performing meridianal therapy on *jitsu*, which accompanies *kyo*, heightens the effect of the total therapy. There are two steps for *jitsu* diagnosis:

1. Diagnosis of *jitsu* in the upper arm

2. Pressure to the *kyo* meridian in the *hara* area

When meridians become *jitsu*, those in the limbs in particular become hard, thick, and resistant. When the healer probes the upper arm, the hardest, most resistant, and thickest line is *jitsu*. Probing is performed on the upper arm rather than the thigh or forearm simply because it is easiest. It must be remembered, however, that because probing *jitsu* in the upper arm is dependent on the healer's sense of touch, it is not difficult to make mistakes. In the upper arm, the thickest and hardest line is the *jitsu* meridian. The yin and yang meridians are often easily mistaken: for instance, if the Lung Meridian is *jitsu*, then the Large Intestine Meridian is also *jitsu*. This means that diagnosis of the *kyo-jitsu* pattern is carried out more accurately by the healer relying on his or her primal sense rather than the sense of touch.

As a prerequisite for diagnosing *jitsu* in the *hara* area, the healer must first of all determine the *kyo* meridians. Then, when continuous pressure is applied to a *kyo* meridian and a *jitsu* meridian at the same time, both are felt as one. This means that when the healer applies continuous pressure to a *kyo* meridian in the *hara* and carries out touch diagnosis on another meridian in the *hara*, the *kyo* and *jitsu* meridians will always be felt as one. As such, the *kyo* meridian is the one determined to correspond to *jitsu* in this way. *Kyo* and *jitsu* meridians can be felt as one when pressed at the same time because at their source, *kyo* and *jitsu* are one and because they are the manifestation of the mutual interrelationship of life.

These methods of *jitsu* diagnosis in the upper arms and in the *hara* area play a complementary role for the inexperienced student of Tao shiatsu. In other words, if a certain degree of *jitsu* is discovered in the upper arm, it can be confirmed in the *hara* area, and conversely, when *jitsu* is diagnosed in the *hara* area, the diagnosis can be confirmed in the upper arms.

Chapter Four

Meridians

Meridians and the Body

Eastern Anatomy

When Western medicine was formally adopted in Japan, those who practiced Oriental medicine were surprised to discover, through Western autopsy, that the position of the internal organs was somewhat different from that indicated in the Classics of Oriental medicine, which they had followed until then. Since the existence of meridians could not be proved through autopsy, practitioners began to wonder if they were not a product of the ancient Chinese imagination. Therapists began to abandon the traditional practices of Oriental medicine and gradually convert to Western medicine. In addition, the government of the Meiji period (1868–1912) passed a bill calling for the eradication of Chinese herbal medicine, and eventually the practice of Oriental therapies became limited to only a select few. (In the West also, natural medicine came to a halt as its practitioners were proclaimed witches, hunted out, and burned.)

As discussed in chapter 1, the concept of *ki* cannot be measured by standards of modern science, and very few Western scientists acknowledge the existence of *ki*. Surprisingly, the existence of meridians has, in recent times, also been called into question among practitioners of therapies categorized as Oriental medicine. At present in Japan, 70 percent of acupuncturists believe they belong to a "science-sect" and practice healing that disregards the existence of meridians. Furthermore, excluding those involved in massage and shiatsu, most therapists of Oriental medicine do not learn about meridians in their training and therefore have slim possibilities of developing meridianal techniques through practical experience. Such trends are a fundamental consequence of the all-too-readily-accepted power of Western civilization in Japan since the Meiji period, which has led many Japanese to become preoccupied with rational thought and scientific analysis. Before the war, "irrational" Japanese mythology was taught to schoolchildren as actual fact. However, because the concept of *ki* and meridians does not fit the Western framework, it has been excluded from curricula on the grounds that it is superstition.

Practitioners of Chinese herbal medicine who had initially thought that meridians were anatomical organs, and not a system of vital functions, were shocked at not being able to discover them through autopsy. But meridians do not exist as anatomical organs; they are a phenomenon of life present only during life and not after death. They are similar to the circulation of blood: as long as an individual is alive, blood flows throughout the body; after death, the blood vessels and the blood serum remain, but the actual blood flow ceases. Blood vessels prove the existence of blood flow, but meridians leave no anatomical remains after death. Therefore, the existence of meridians was initially refuted because it could not be proved objectively or by analytical techniques. Masunaga describes meridians as the protoplasm that flows through the cells. This flow only exists while a person is alive and stops with death. Similarly, because meridians are the currents of the *ki* of life, no trace of them remains after death.

The anatomical organs that make up our physical structures and remain even after death are of course essential to life. But they are not life itself; they are nothing more than tools that support the living body. Meridians are much closer to the essence of life than physical organs. Similarly, although the existence of pleasure and displeasure cannot be proven objectively, they are also considered to be the essence of life and, throughout life, living creatures avoid displeasure and seek pleasure. Meridians are more than the manifestation of life; they contain and distribute the vitality that controls the functions of all the anatomical organs. As such, it is far more correct to perceive death as the time when meridianal circulation stops, and therefore the functions of life stop, than to suppose that meridians merely disappear after death. It may be said, therefore, that the essence of life is energy and not the physical structures of the body.

Western Diagnosis in Oriental Medicine

Once the concept of meridians is excluded from therapeutic methods such as shiatsu and acupuncture, these practices can no longer be categorized as Oriental medicine. If practitioners of shiatsu, acupuncture, and moxibustion cannot perform diagnosis through meridians, the only method of diagnosis is categorizing illness—the method employed by Western medicine. Therapeutic methods based on categorizing illness and those based on meridianal diagnosis are born from completely different cultures and medical systems. Masunaga proposes that whether a method of treatment is worthy of being called medicine depends on the system of diagnosis it uses. Even a highly effective healing method cannot be called a comprehensive discipline if it is not based on an appropriate system of diagnosis. Acceptance of the Western system means that such shiatsu and acupuncture therapists do not rely on their own methods of diagnosis but use the diagnostic method provided by Western medicine. This ultimately means that they are forced to rely on Western medicine to decide on therapy. It is questionable, therefore, whether such practitioners can even be called doctors, because a healer unable to make a decision on therapy cannot be responsible for treatment.

Systems of diagnosis and treatment vary according to the cultures from which they originate. Diagnosis is not simply limited to objective recognition of conditions of illness, as is the case in Western medicine. The Oriental perspective on diagnosis (such as *sho*, the diagnosis of the *kyo-jitsu* pattern), allows a choice of therapy designed for each individual patient. (Individual diagnosis may also exist in healing practices carried out by shamans in "primitive" societies.) A form of therapy does not function as an act of medical treatment unless it relies on diagnosis based on the same system, and treatment performed without diagnosis is nothing more than an unofficial form of amateur therapy.

The Primal Sense

Meridians are related to invisible life, and their existence cannot be proved anatomically. The essence of life can only be perceived by actual sensations and not by the intellectualization of objective distinctions between the self and others. What is visible, and therefore perceived by conscious analysis, is an extremely small portion of existence. In a person's life, the most important things are love and pleasure, freedom and virtue, over and above position and honor: all intangibles. In fact, these invisible attributes actually enable the materialization of what is visible. Meridians form the background of the visible anatomical organs and are at the source of all vital functions. When studying meridians, beginners understandably follow the lines on a diagram to learn their positions. However, because meridians characteristically exist in constant circulation, they cannot be considered fixed in any one position. Novices often make the mistake of trying to understand the physical position of meridians in the body. Unless healers respond to the movement of meridians, they cannot truly cure the disorders. Therefore, in order to carry out correct meridianal diagnosis and administer appropriate treatment, the healer's receptivity must be heightened to the extent that he or she is able to respond to the state of meridianal circulation.

According to one practitioner of acupuncture, a fourteen-year-old patient who had never heard of meridians was able to clearly see and almost accurately trace the meridianal lines on the surface of the body. As the years passed, however, her extraordinary ability began to diminish and eventually disappeared. This ability is by no means unique. As human beings, in order to function within our social environment, we develop a sense of discrimination that weakens our primal senses. An explanation for the loss of this patient's ability to feel the meridians may be that the emergence of her self-consciousness suppressed her primal sensitivity to *ki*.

What is necessary for the recognition of meridians is not a superior intelligence or a keen sense of touch (the latter belongs in the realm of the discriminatory senses) but a simple, inarticulate empathy, which ultimately means feeling another's pain and joy as one's own—one indication of a heightened primal sense. The great teacher Christ preached that unless people became "like children" they would not enter heaven. Healers, too, cannot detect meridians unless they have the innocence of a child. Because we live in a competitive society that inclines toward yang, we are brought up on the idea that we must always be one step ahead of the next person. This fosters a strong sense of distinction between the self and others, suppressing the primal sense and dulling our sensitivity to life and the pain and suffering of others. Those who are indifferent to others have no difficulty in living in present-day society, although their potential to experience the pleasures of life is diminished. The actual sensations of life can only be attained through a mind that is able to accept contrast but does not distinguish between the self and others. Those who have a heightened sense of empathy toward others are also able to savor the pleasures of life instead of its bitterness and hardships. Criminals who injure or kill others are not fundamentally evil but have weakened vital senses, lacking empathy toward the lives of others and the power to imagine their pain and suffering.

People who live in modern society generally have weak imaginations. This may be because fundamental belief in mythology has been shattered by scientific theory. For instance, most Japanese used to believe the moon to be a

place where rabbits lived. However, scientific discoveries and space explora-
tion have rendered the moon a bleak place, and people no longer believe the
myth they once naturally saw there. The influence of science and the increasing disregard for the spirituality of mythology have generated an ideology
that only values what is visible and what can be understood objectively. According to the Western psychologist Jung, UFOs are a new myth for modern
people who have lost their belief in traditional myth. In other words, UFOs
are a modern myth in scientific disguise.

In ancient times, people's imaginative powers allowed them to see an
abundance of gods behind all nature, which is not unrelated to the fact that
their primal sense was, as yet, unsuppressed. Similarly, because people believed in nature, they also believed in reincarnation—the cycle of death, re-
birth, and life after death. Modern people cannot believe in a world after
death because modern trends are founded on materialism and the people
lack the imagination to envision a world after death. Our primal sense is also
essential for the understanding of meridians and may be developed through
Oriental disciplinary training. When our primal sense develops, we are able
to recognize the existence of meridians, and we are awakened to a deeply
rooted consciousness enabling us to feel another's life as though it were our
own. When this takes place, we are, for instance, able to feel the life of an in-
sect as our own life and the comfort of an infant in its mother's arms as our
own comfort. All our responses to life are heightened and it becomes difficult
for us to inflict pain or injury on others, even insects.

Our increasing empathy toward others does not mean that we lose our
own ego; rather, while maintaining our own self-consciousness, we sense the
world as one entity deep within that consciousness. In Buddhism, this wisdom, without antagonism, is called *indiscrete wisdom*, and the discerning in-
tellect that uses rational thought is called *worldly wisdom* (these two are
always kept separate). What allows recognition of the meridians is very similar to indiscrete wisdom. Furthermore, if one does not have a heightened
sense for life, no amount of concentration will reveal the meridians. It is similar to being unable to appreciate the beauty of a painting unless one has a
mind that can comprehend that beauty. In other words, unless one has the
innocence of a child, one cannot see meridians.

In ancient times, people were not restricted by the modern ego that con-
fines us today. For example, because our ancestors had a heightened sensitivity toward nature, they were able to predict changes in climatic conditions.
It is thought that the ancient Chinese were able to discover meridians be-

cause of their heightened primal sense and their receptivity to the *ki* of life. The various mental and physical disciplinary training methods of martial arts, meditation, yoga, and *sendo* all aim to heighten a person's primal sense. The increasing interest in these disciplines is perhaps a natural reaction to the weakening of the primal sense that is caused by a materialistic lifestyle. It is for the same reason that people are turning to shiatsu as a form of therapy.

Six, Twelve, and Twenty-Four Meridians

Meridians Noted in the Classics

The Classics mention only six meridians in each arm and leg but Masunaga's diagrams show twelve meridians throughout the body. My work proposes twice as many meridians. Since the concept of twelve meridians throughout the body was not noted in the Classics, those who base their therapy on the traditional theory of meridians have had difficulty accepting it. Masunaga explains the developments that led to the discovery of the twelve meridians as follows:

> *I began to understand that meridians existed in parts of the body not mentioned in the Classics by recognizing the response pattern of each patient's state of illness and perceiving that this response pattern corresponded to an equal response in the whole body. Thus I identified meridian lines not noted in the Classics and, by treating many different patients, gradually defined this technique through the process of developing effective cures for meridianal disorders.[1]*

Masunaga also notes that meridians in the Classics were conveniently simplified according to the practices of acupuncture and moxibustion. One reason for this was that at the time that meridians were reported in the Clas-

---

1. Shizuto Masunaga, *Keiraku to Shiatsu* [in Japanese] (Yokosuka: Ido no Nihonsha, 1983).

sics, the main focus of therapy was already moving away from the manual technique. The medical knowledge that had, until then, been handed down by mere novices to their colleagues was changed to suit the classroom environment. In order to train a large number of students at a time, the positions of the meridians were clearly defined and the number of *tsubo* was established at around 360. However, because *tsubo* are phenomena of changeable life, it is unnatural to limit their number. Therapies of Oriental medicine focus on *ki*, the background of what is physically visible. Therefore students had to begin developing a sense toward *ki* that allowed them to discover the *tsubo* on which they were to perform therapy. Formalized training of large numbers of students through mass education probably necessitated even more conveniences than merely naming the acupuncture points and establishing their anatomical position.

Furthermore, acupuncture and moxibustion were not considered safe because they caused a degree of injury to the body (the Classics note in detail how many days it takes for a person to die after a needle has been inserted in certain points of the body). The Classics state that the acupuncture points were perceived as being anatomically positioned in order to avoid the dangers ensuing from acupuncture. Once the acupuncture points were established, the meridians were no longer of any great importance. This is because, once the healer has determined the meridians as being either *kyo* or *jitsu* through pulse diagnosis, treatment is then carried out on the appropriate acupuncture points and the healer no longer needs to regard the meridians as lines. Meridians were traditionally described as lines connecting the acupuncture points rather than as currents of true vitality. As such, limiting them to six on each arm and leg was not at all difficult. Also, traditional theory proposes that the direction of the meridians switches back and forth and, after turning at right angles, once again follows a straight line. This is said to indicate that meridians that are two lines at their source become one.

Evidence for Twelve Meridians

It is thought that the diagrams of meridians recorded in the Classics are an abbreviation of what may have existed earlier, and that the twelve meridians throughout the body reported by Masunaga is a review of the Classical record. The theory of the twelve meridians was confirmed by Masunaga's own clinical experience. However, it is not generally accepted by practitioners of acupuncture and moxibustion, who repeatedly asked Masunaga to explain his findings of those meridians not mentioned in the Classics.

There is only one answer to the multitude of questions from those who do not accept Masunaga's findings. Naturally, the ultimate proof that twelve meridians circulate throughout the body can be established by one's own personal clinical experience. There is, however, a much more effective method of proving this, which is also very useful for the study of meridianal therapy: application of the rule in meridianal treatment that states that when a healer applies pressure to two points of the same meridian, the two points should be felt as one. For instance, when continuous pressure is applied to the Triple Heater *tsubo* on the back of the hand and on the top of the foot simultaneously (the latter *tsubo* is not noted in the Classics), after a few seconds, the patient no longer feels the pressure on two points of his or her body but begins to feel it as one. In contrast, if pressure is applied to the Triple Heater *tsubo* on the back of the hand and to the Gall Bladder Meridian on the top of the foot simultaneously, the patient will feel the pressure as on two separate points. (Of course, some people have a strong sense of conscious discrimination and are therefore weak in sensing the meridians. Such people are inappropriate for this experiment.)

In my opinion, there is not much point in trying to go further to prove the theory of the twelve meridians. Therefore, I do not intend to force this theory on those therapists who believe in, and practice healing through, the use of the traditional meridians. If this theory has any significance, through its use, students can learn about the correct meridians and their patients will receive appropriate meridianal treatment. The most important thing in medicine is not proving a theory but contributing to a person's health through selection of the most effective form of therapy.

The Discovery of the Twenty-Four Meridians

At first, I never considered the possibility of the existence of more meridians than the twelve proposed by Masunaga's meridian chart.[2] However, I noticed an increase in the number of patients who did not heal through the use

---

2. Shizuto Masunaga, *Shiatsu Keiraku Zu* [in Japanese] (Tokyo: Iokai Shiatsu Institute, 1983).

of the meridians noted in the existing diagrams. Initially, these were patients with back complaints. In Masunaga's Shiatsu Meridian Chart, only the Small Intestine, Triple Heater, and Gall Bladder Meridians run on the back, omitting the Bladder Meridian. But I realized that the source of back complaints was not necessarily in any one of these meridians and, in diagnosing the *kyo-jitsu* pattern, I saw many cases where disorders in the lungs and small intestine were completely inconsistent with symptoms and diagnostic conclusions. Furthermore, meridians did not always indicate the ailing part of the body. These inconsistencies led me to consider the possible existence of meridians other than those indicated in Masunaga's chart.

In much the same way, I believe, that Masunaga discovered the twelve meridians throughout the body, I became aware that applying pressure to certain *tsubo* resulted in a response pattern corresponding with the response in the whole body. In other words, the meridians corresponding to the ailing part of the body were confirmed, based on the patient's response. This was consistent with all diagnostic conclusions, and patients with back problems that had, until then, been difficult to treat showed signs of recovery. By becoming aware of the existence of twenty-four meridians circulating throughout the body that function in the same way as Masunaga's twelve meridians based on the traditional theory, I was able to answer some of Masunaga's own questions, such as: "until now, diagrams of meridians have been somewhat unclear as to the type of therapy to administer in cases where the healer feels that therapy is necessary but the symptoms are present in a part of the body where there are no acupuncture points or meridians" and "when the response pattern corresponds with a response in the whole body, how is it possible to acknowledge the pattern in meridianal flow even in parts of the body not noted in the classics?"[3]

Since meridians are the currents of life, it is inconceivable that they should stop in any one place. Therefore, the theory of only six meridians in each arm and leg does not seem feasible. It is also unnatural to consider that the meridians in the legs run up the thigh and stop at the crotch, as is implied by Masunaga's theory. The theory of twenty-four meridians proposes that the meridians in the legs do not stop at the crotch but rise up to the back across the buttocks and connect with all the meridians shown in Masunaga's Shia-

---

3. Shizuto Masunaga, *Setshin no Tebiki* [in Japanese] (Tokyo: Iokai Shiatsu Institute, 1983).

tsu Meridian Chart. In fact there are twelve meridians on each side of the back. In the diagram of the twelve meridians throughout the body, there are twelve lines in the arms and legs and each meridian has its own direction. It has also been confirmed through clinical experience that meridians in the arms and legs flow in pairs.

Another important discovery through therapy has been that the Conception and Governor Vessels exist in the arms and legs as well as in the back region. In previous diagrams of meridians, these vessels were only shown to exist in the center on the front and back of the body. Therefore, there was no appropriate means of therapy for patients with a *kyo* condition of these vessels. However, it has since become possible to administer effective therapy even for this type of condition through the use of the meridians in the arms and legs.

The Classics note an unorthodox meridian running around the waist. In fact, each meridian has several branches that form a horizontal network throughout the body. Depending on the particular case, clinically, symptoms and *tsubo* may be present at the intersections of the *kyo* meridians throughout the body. This may be used to indicate the point where therapy is to be administered. When *kyo* symptoms become chronic, they appear first in the *kyo* meridians and the sub-meridians. Then, if they are not treated, they appear in the meridians running horizontally throughout the body and the Spiral Meridian.

The meridians in the back region are of great clinical importance. The sub-meridians in the hands and feet generally manifest symptoms in cases where the disorder has advanced to abnormal stages. I believe that Masunaga knew more about the existence of meridians in the back region than what he indicated in *Keiraku to Shiatsu*. He discovered the twelve meridians in the whole body and had such a keen sense for meridians that there is no reason to think he did not know about the existence of the others. Perhaps he did not include the back-region meridians in his twelve-meridian theory because they were unnecessary for treating conditions existing at that time. In Masunaga's time, most patients presented *jitsu* symptoms, and it was sufficient to carry out therapy using only the meridians in the legs and arms. In other words, because the sources of the symptoms of back and neck ailments were largely *jitsu*, it was possible to provide relief with only a few minutes of strong pressure to the *kyo* meridians in the arms and legs. Because at that particular time, effective treatment was possible even without using the meridians in the back region, omitting them had no therapeutic effect. (Masunaga actually demonstrated this type of therapy on patients at lectures and surprised all his students, including me. When I first began to deliver my own lectures, I demonstrated these same methods and was able to easily relieve a *jitsu* symptom with a *kyo* treatment in front of those watching.) Indeed, the six meridians noted in the Classics provided sufficiently effective therapy for those particular times.

In modern times, however, effective treatment cannot be provided without considering all twenty-four meridians throughout the body. This is because we have entered a yin period, in which the patient's symptoms tend to be directed inward. In the yang period, the resolutions of the materialist world are carried out through science, and in the yin period, resolutions become inherently more spiritual. Meridians, too, belong to the world of yin and at present there is a need to urge therapy for patients with *kyo* symptoms. Therefore, recognition of twenty-four meridians flowing throughout the body is essential.

The *Kyo-Jitsu* Pattern in the Meridians

The Role of Each Meridian

In diagrams, because meridians run along the surface of the body, they seem to belong in the realm of the physical. However, as we come to see that all mental and physical functions are subject to meridians, we realize that meridians are inextricably bound with the life of the universe. From the understanding of the human body as a miniature universe is born an awareness of the Eastern view of life: the part is equal to the whole. Disorders in *ki*, the vital force of the universe and therefore of the mind and body, are manifested as *kyo-jitsu* patterns in the meridians.

Kyo-jitsu patterns are patterns of disorder and disharmony. However, this does not mean that they can be measured or that their normal state can be compared to an abnormal state. This differs from Western diagnostic methods, which calculate what is normal or abnormal. The *kyo-jitsu* pattern in the meridians is not an indication of whether one patient has a disorder compa-rable to that of other patients; it is a diagnosis that identifies disorders in *ki*. Although the *kyo-jitsu* pattern is not an indication of illness in itself, extremes in one or the other develop into illness. The *kyo-jitsu* pattern is as essential to life as the opposition of yin and yang. *Kyo* is a deficiency or a yearning. All bodies create desires for what is lacking (for instance, the desire for food when one is hungry results in the action of eating). *Jitsu* is the concentration of energy essential for action. The action of someone picking something up, for instance, creates a *jitsu* condition because certain muscles are tightened and employed. In other words, *jitsu* is the concentration of energy essential for performing an act in order to fulfill a desire (*kyo*). From this point of view, we may learn to understand why *kyo-jitsu* disorders occur in the body and what treatments can be used.

As all life functions are carried out by *kyo-jitsu* patterns, ultimately, after the function has been completed, it is natural for the body to return to a state of rest. (Even animals return to a state of rest after performing a function.) However, since humans are not easily satisfied, we continue to think about a task even after it is completed. Disorders in the *kyo-jitsu* pattern are generat-ed when a certain task occupies our mind even when we are not actually per-forming that task. If a desire (*kyo*) is not fulfilled even after a task has been completed, a disorder in *ki* sets in and creates an *induration* (*jitsu*). In such cases, regardless of how much shiatsu pressure is applied to the area, the *jit-su* induration cannot be dissolved. Even if the disorder seems to be relieved during therapy, it returns later and manifests more severe symptoms than before. This is because it is created by a concentration of energy (*ki*) for the purpose of fulfilling the initial desire.

When the *kyo-jitsu* disorder deepens and settles in, it may manifest vari-ous symptoms. Conversely, when the disorder resolves and the pattern is in constant change, the person is healthy. Likewise nature and life are in con-stant change, and fixation means death. Since the various disciplinary meth-ods of the East aim to reach a flexibility of the mind and body that can respond to all changes (chapter 2), in the psychological sense, they are said to be able to surpass death.

Lung and Large Intestine

The Lung Meridian is so closely related to the breath that when pressure is applied to this meridian, the breath deepens. Patients with *kyo* Lung Meridians have increased markedly in recent times. This is probably because people react to air pollution by avoiding deep inhalation. The Lung *kyo* pattern is indicated by shallow breathing and poor oxygen supply. The Lung Meridian also runs along the thumbs. Clenching one's fists around the thumbs, therefore, creates difficulties for deep inhalation. People with Lung *kyo* have a characteristic tendency to lean forward. This posture is the most comfortable because the first, second, and third thoracic vertebrae have receded (they are also controlled by the Lung Meridian), and the body unavoidably leans forward. This posture may also be a reaction to the subconscious need to protect the *kyo* meridian in the *hara* area. However, when the body leans forward, it becomes difficult to inhale deeply and, naturally, the supply of oxygen deteriorates.

The Lung Meridian expands when one pushes out the chest in order to inhale deeply. This is indicative of the close relationship between posture and physiological functions: when one adopts a certain posture, the meridians responsible for the physiological function expand. First, the meridians expand through the movement of *ki* and physiological functions are performed by adopting a posture in response to the meridians. Second, the posture adopted through the expansion and contraction of the meridians is also closely related to psychological functions. For instance, pushing out one's chest when inhaling deeply stimulates feelings of liberation, whereas leaning forward hinders breathing and creates feelings of physical handicap. There are many reasons in modern times for the increased number of people with Lung *kyo*. One reason is the demands of the transition into the yin phase, in which the focus is on internal spirituality rather than external materialism, making people become more introspective (chapter 3).

One Lung *kyo* patient in my own clinical experience was a man in his late thirties with cerebral palsy who, despite his disability, had a normal occupation and was able to lead a relatively normal life. His physical handicaps were that his head sat badly and his posture and walk were awkward, because his first, second, and third thoracic vertebrae were misaligned so much that they did not seem to be correctable. Because the Lung Meridian in the back region had not yet been discovered, as treatment (apart from basic whole-body shiatsu), I supplemented the Lung Meridian in the arms and legs. Surprisingly, although I hardly even touched his spinal column, the misaligned vertebrae gradually began to correct themselves, which in turn improved his posture, the position of his head, and his walk. Because the whole body is essentially connected through the meridians, in this case, meridianal treatment on the legs and arms resulted in changes in other parts of the body.

The Classics state that the whites of the eyes belong to the Lung Meridian, but perhaps this is related to the fact that the eye consumes a large amount of oxygen. The Lung Meridian is closely connected with deep inhalation. The *kyo* pattern of the Lung Meridian and both *kyo* and *jitsu* patterns of the Large Intestine Meridian are common, but the Lung *jitsu* pattern, which hinders breathing, is very rare. Because the Lung and the Large Intestine Meridians have the yin-yang relationship, whenever the Lung is *kyo*, the Large Intestine is also *kyo*. The Lung Meridian is never *kyo* when the Large Intestine Meridian is *jitsu*. Therefore at present, since there are many Lung *kyo* patients, there are also many Large Intestine *kyo* patients. In many cases, colds and sore throats are caused by a *kyo* condition in the Large Intestine. At such times, patients may relieve the discomfort themselves with shiatsu to the Large Intestine Meridian in the forearm. Constipation is also due to the Large Intestine becoming *kyo*, which weakens one's power to eliminate. In such cases, shiatsu to the Large Intestine Meridian in the legs is very effective. Diarrhea is also caused by Gall Bladder *kyo* (inability to digest fats) or Stomach *kyo*.

For each organ to perform its individual vital function, it must maintain a constant exchange of energy with other organs. The Lung and Large Intestine Meridians function within this vital exchange, and organs such as the breathing apparatus and skin belong to the Lung and Large Intestine Meridian system. The *kyo* pattern of the Large Intestine Meridian is generally caused by the constant craving for yin products such as coffee and spicy foods, which cause *ki* to rise. People who are prone to this condition generally tend to have a weakening of the throat and skin that gets infected easily. The Lung Meridian expands when people embrace one another; therefore, this meridian has a psychological effect on the exchange between the self and others and is closely related to feelings of liberation and acceptance. The Large Intestine Meridian is responsible for the function of expelling excretions to the outside. Therefore, psychologically, it is closely related to self-expression—expressing externally what one feels internally. The basic vocal functions of singing and speaking are also carried out by the Large Intestine Meridian, which controls throat vibrations. Expressions such as writing and drawing rely on the Large Intestine Meridian in the arms. A *jitsu* pattern is generated in the Large Intestine Meridian when one is unable to express oneself verbally, causing frequent sighing in order to expel inner thoughts. Conversely, the *kyo* pattern of the Large Intestine Meridian is manifested as a state where willful expression is lost.

Stomach and Spleen

Stomach *kyo* patients are considerably fewer than Stomach *jitsu* patients. One reason for this is the absence of serious symptoms manifested by the Stomach *kyo* pattern, which is actually far more common than Stomach *jitsu* because it is caused by excess food and drink. The Stomach Meridian runs along the front of the legs, and when this meridian becomes *jitsu*, it cannot expand. Also, because the muscles are among the organs belonging to the Stomach Meridian, the Stomach *jitsu* pattern may manifest muscular pain. Painful joints, however, are often caused by the *jitsu* pattern of the Gall Bladder Meridian, which governs the joints throughout the body.

The most natural expression of the *kyo-jitsu* disorder is when a person's stomach is empty (Stomach *kyo*) and when it is full (Stomach *jitsu*). Where there is a tendency toward overeating, a disorder settles in and the stomach is unable to return to its normal state. The Stomach Meridian includes not only the stomach organ itself but all organs of the alimentary canal, beginning with the mouth and including all the organs of digestion, the muscles, and the breasts. Traditionally, the function of the Stomach Meridian was said to be "accepting internally those things that came from the outside world." Psychologically, this means being able to accept one's immediate environment. Therefore, symptoms such as children's loss of appetite, characteristic of Stomach *kyo*, are more an expression of difficulty in accepting one's home environment than the loss of the desire for food. Generally, those who suffer from Stomach *kyo* complain of gastric imbalance and characteristically drink a lot of fluids with their meals, because this condition decreases the secretion of saliva and the energy to accept things from the outside. The *kyo* pattern of the Gall Bladder and Triple Heater Meridians causes the same feeling of gastric imbalance. For instance, in the case of Gall Bladder *kyo*, the inability to digest fats caused by a decrease in the secretion of bile manifests feelings of gastric imbalance. The Gall Bladder *kyo* pattern is often caused by a high intake of foods that require detoxification, such as white sugar and chemical additives. The Triple Heater *kyo* pattern is caused by over-sensitivity of the mucous membrane of the stomach. Furthermore, gastric ulcers are often manifested by Heart *kyo* (ulceration of the cardiac region) or Heart Constrictor *kyo* (ulceration of the pyloric region).

The Spleen *kyo* pattern is more common than the Stomach *kyo* pattern. As can be seen in the diagram (Figure 4.7), the Spleen Meridian runs down from the temple area toward the legs. Because its fundamental functions have to do with digestion, the Spleen Meridian controls the secretion of digestive juices, such as saliva and gastric juices. Expansion and contraction of the Spleen Meridian, which runs down the cheeks, take place through the action of chewing, which stimulates the secretion of saliva, the first step of digestion. The Spleen Meridian in the abdominal area is positioned around the navel and corresponds to the solar plexus, also positioned in this region and known as the "second brain."

The Spleen Meridian also includes the knees and ankles, which are the only joints not positioned on the Liver and Gall Bladder Meridians. Therefore, people who have weak knees often have Spleen *kyo*. (The healer must be cautious, however, because painful knee joints may be due to the *kyo* pattern of the Spleen, Bladder, or Lungs and can actually improve without any kind of treatment at all.) In one case a woman complained of difficulty in walking and extending her knees because of a fall she sustained some years previously. Observing her *hara* area, I saw that her condition was Spleen *kyo*. I advised her that if she chewed well, she would soon be able to extend her knees. One month later, she came back to tell me that she had been chewing sugarless gum and had gradually regained the ability to bend her knees and her walking had improved. The action of chewing heightens the function of the Spleen Meridian. The Spleen Meridian also controls the brain, and the Japanese saying that chewing fosters intelligence was born from the fact that chewing heightens the function of this meridian. (Also, the Spleen Meridian controls the spleen as well as the pancreas; therefore, diabetes, which is caused by a deficiency of the insulin secreted from the Langerhans islet of the pancreas, exhibits the *kyo-jitsu* pattern in the Spleen Meridian.)

Heart and Small Intestine

According to the Five Color Method of Classification in Chinese medicine, the Heart and Small Intestine Meridians are red. This is probably because they are closely related to the blood and the blood vessels. According to Masunaga, the main functions of these meridians are *conversion* and *regulation*. The Small Intestine Meridian *regulates* the whole body through the blood vessels and *converts* food taken in and digested through the stomach and spleen into blood, absorbing the food as nutrition. Indications of the *kyo* pattern in the Small Intestine are insufficient blood flow caused by the constriction of the blood vessels, irregularity in the menstrual cycle, and feeling cold, caused by poor circulation in the legs. (When shiatsu therapy is administered to *kyo* Small Intestine Meridians, patients comment that somehow their legs become warm.)

When a bruise appears after a blow, strong pressure to the Small Intestine Meridian in the arms and legs (particularly on the opposite side of the affected area) is very effective. When the healer applies this kind of pressure immediately after the bruise has formed, patients get the surprise of seeing it disappear before their very eyes. This was the case when I administered shiatsu to the Small Intestine Meridian of a child who had fallen and sustained bruises while practicing aikido. The *kyo* pattern of the Small Intestine is also common after sprains; however, in most cases, the *kyo* pattern of the Small Intestine actually preceded the sprain. In other words, the pre-existing *kyo* pattern of the Small Intestine caused the sprain rather than the other way around.

Kyo is yin, a negative force, and *kyo* meridians have the function of drawing increasingly inward. People who are yin and negative have the tendency to take advantage of others. Even if a person is rational, because they have a void in their mind, they are drawn in by people who have negative, yin characteristics. Therefore, it is essential to unite the mind with the body in daily life so as not to create a void in the mind. Sprains are caused by drawing the *kyo* meridians into places that have been emptied of *ki*. Immediately after a sprain has been sustained, the Small Intestine becomes *kyo*; if this condition is allowed to continue for several days, it results in Lung *kyo* and Gall Bladder *jitsu*. The latter is indicative of the fact that the sprain has caused all the joints in the body to become stiff.

One high school student came to me complaining of a stiff shoulder, which she had endured for some years. Diagnosis revealed that she was Heart *kyo* and Gall Bladder *jitsu*. I asked whether she had been involved in some sort of accident and she replied that she had been hit by a car in her early teens. When I suggested that this was the reason for her stiff shoulder, she was reluctant to accept my diagnosis because the accident had not been serious. I applied pressure to the stiff area (Gall Bladder *jitsu*) and she was surprised to learn that her stiffness could be relieved by pressure to the pit of her abdomen (the Heart *kyo* pattern in the *hara*). After performing shiatsu on the Heart Meridian in the arms and legs, I treated the Gall Bladder *jitsu* with the *sha* method and when, lastly, I corrected the third and fourth thoracic vertebrae, her stiffness was relieved.

A typical complaint caused by Small Intestine *kyo* is hernia of the intervertebral disk, commonly called a slipped disk. This is often caused by the *kyo* pattern of the Small Intestine Meridian in the *hara* area being drawn in, and the misalignment of the first and second lumbar vertebrae. Recently, however, more and more intervertebral hernias have been caused by Bladder *kyo* or Lung *kyo*. This problem cannot be corrected effectively through Masunaga's theory of twelve meridians throughout the body, and it is therefore essential to consider the new proposition of the twenty-four meridians throughout the body.

As mentioned above, the Small Intestine Meridian converts food products taken into the body from the outside into blood. The Heart Meridian also has the function of regulating and converting. The heart is the source of the imagination, which changes external stimulation into internal images and understanding. Sustaining a shock or suffering psychological stress over an extended period of time changes one's mental condition into *kyo*. This is because the external stimulus received by the Heart Meridian is so strong that the Heart Meridian is weakened by the shock. There are many psychiatric patients with *kyo* condition of the Heart Meridian who are overwhelmed by hallucinations and delusions created by their own subconscious and are unable to conceptualize the outside world correctly.

The tongue is one of the organs positioned along the heart meridian. Masunaga explains that his patients who have speech impediments also present Heart *kyo*. Because I have never diagnosed this type of patient in my own clinical experience, I cannot comment on this condition.

Kidney and Bladder

In the Theory of the Five Elements of Yin and Yang, the Kidney and Bladder Meridians belong in the realm of water. They perform the functions of urine production and fluid excretion. The Kidney Meridian is the source of vigor and is said to control resistance to stress and volition. In particular, because the Kidney Meridian in the *hara* area includes the *tanden* (chapter 1), when it becomes *kyo*, the individual loses the ability to persist in tasks and the sense of individuality begins to become unstable. Furthermore, this meridian is closely related to internal secretions such as that of the sex hormones. Sexual excess causes a *kyo* condition of the Kidney Meridian, which indicates exhaustion of one's sexual vigor.

The *jitsu* pattern of the Kidney Meridian has been predominant in recent times. There are two possible reasons for this. One is the psychological stress of living in modern society, and the other is poor dietary habits. For instance, one's Kidney Meridian may become *jitsu* only thirty minutes after one drinks coffee. Coffee causes a severe constriction of this meridian that is very easy to recognize in the arms and legs. This is because caffeine causes unnecessary secretion of adrenaline, which distorts the hormonal balance. Cakes, sweets, and other foods made from refined white sugar also cause Kidney and Bladder *jitsu*, not as quickly as coffee but more deeply. White sugar also causes a rapid increase in the blood sugar level and, in order to rectify this increase, the body secretes hormones that lower the blood sugar to below normal levels, once again creating a desire for sweets. While this process is repeated, hormonal balance is disrupted and the Kidney Meridian becomes *jitsu*. When hormonal imbalance continues, it affects the midbrain, resulting in irregularity of the autonomic nerves, which causes the *jitsu* condition of the Kidney to move to the Bladder. What coffee and white sugar have in common is that soon after consumption they alleviate fatigue and stimulate a feeling of excitement. However, several hours later, the feeling of fatigue returns and with it the craving for more stimulation by these foods.

Traditional theory holds that the *ki* of the universe enters the body via the Kidney Meridian, which is closely related to longevity and aging. The Classics also note that the state of the *ki* of the Kidney Meridian differs with age, thereby determining the aging process. This may be why Taoists, who practiced disciplines to promote the health of the kidneys, were able to prolong their lives. Indeed, the parts of the body that belong to the Kidney Meridian —the hair, the bones, the teeth, and the pupils of the eyes—all deteriorate with a person's age. Aging actually begins with the weakening of the Kidney Meridian and, as a result, the physical organs also weaken. The disciplinary methods used by the Chinese, who are said to have the potential for perennial youth, have one aim without exception: concentrating on the abdominal *tanden* in order to strengthen it. Strengthening the abdominal *tanden* also strengthens the Kidney Meridian—the center of *ki*—and enriches *ki* throughout the body. If the Kidney Meridian is always kept in perfect condition and its *ki* continues to be heightened, the aging process may be controlled.

Bladder *kyo* and Bladder *jitsu* are both common conditions. When the Bladder becomes *kyo*, the most common complaints are urinary weakness and insomnia. Insomnia is also caused by Bladder *jitsu*, in which case it occurs because stress in the sympathetic nerves cannot be relieved. This kind of insomnia is not as serious as that caused by Bladder *kyo*, in which the nerves become oversensitive and one can be awakened by the slightest sound. For some reason Bladder *kyo* causing sleep disturbances is often a result of personal stress. The Bladder Meridian is also responsible for preparing the mind and body for a forthcoming action. Therefore, when the Bladder becomes *kyo*, it hinders the functions between one action and the next. This is also related to the fact that the function of the sympathetic nerves has slowed down. One of the organs positioned on the Bladder Meridian is the womb, and female sterility and other gynecological problems are often caused by Bladder *kyo*. In particular, women who are sterile also have characteristic symptoms of severe stiffness of the hips, recession of the sacral vertebrae, or chills. In such cases, a beneficial therapy is to relieve the stiffness caused by the *kyo* condition of the Bladder Meridian in the back and lower back area.

As mentioned earlier, Bladder *jitsu* indicates a condition where stress in the sympathetic nerves cannot be relieved. Also, because the Bladder Meridian is responsible for preparation for a forthcoming action, Bladder *jitsu* is prevalent in those who are under constant pressure to always be on schedule, making constant demands on their body in order to prepare for endless forthcoming tasks.

Heart Constrictor and Triple Heater

The Heart Constrictor Meridian is a yin meridian that controls the main blood vessels such as the aorta and coronary arteries. The Triple Heater, a yang meridian, controls the peripheral circulation (circulation near the surface of the body) and body fluids. The skin, serous membranes, and mucous membranes are positioned on this meridian. The Triple Heater is divided into Upper, Middle, and Lower levels. The Upper is responsible for membranes from the chest to the brain, the Middle for the membranes from the navel to the greater omentum, and the Lower for the lower abdominal and intestinal membranes and the membranes of the womb.

The symptoms of the *kyo* pattern of the Heart Constrictor Meridian are palpitations and abnormal blood pressure, mental vagueness through lack of circulation, and Ménière's syndrome. An interesting clinical example of this condition was presented by a patient who was unable to open his mouth after having fallen from a cherry tree. Visual diagnosis revealed the *kyo* pattern in the Heart Constrictor, and only three minutes after I applied shiatsu to his *hara* area, he was able to open his mouth wide. The Heart Constrictor had probably become *kyo* because of the shock of falling from the tree. Shock causes a *kyo* condition of the Heart, which leads to Heart Constrictor *kyo* if it goes untreated. The Heart Constrictor *kyo* pattern is often a cause of Basedow's disease, and Masunaga explains that this may be due to strong subconscious fears of death. Those with this *kyo* pattern, which results in symptoms such as palpitations, adopt a physical posture that reveals feelings of subconscious fear.

Because the Triple Heater Meridian controls peripheral circulation, when the Triple Heater becomes *kyo*, the body becomes cold. When it is cold, we instinctively hug our own body and rub our arms: an unconscious action to stimulate the Triple Heater Meridian in the upper arms, which improves peripheral circulation and warms the body. The basic function of the Triple Heater Meridian is adaptation to the outside world, physical defense, and protection. Actions such as unconsciously raising the hands to protect oneself from being hit by a flying object are performed by the expansion of the Triple Heater Meridian. Actions such as manipulation of the steering wheel while driving a car are also functions of this meridian. The typical patterns of disorder caused by whiplash injury in car accidents are Triple Heater *jitsu*, caused by instinctively grasping the steering wheel to protect the body, and Small Intestine *kyo*, caused by the shock of the accident. Also, in the first stages of neurosis, because the ability to adapt to the outside world is weakened, the pattern of the Triple Heater is *kyo*. The *jitsu* pattern of the Triple Heater indicates *overconformity*. This means that when a person is overly aware of others in his or her immediate environment, the Triple Heater becomes excessively *jitsu* and often such people have difficulty in moving their head.

The cause of allergies has less to do with allergens than with the weakening of the Triple Heater Meridian. When the Triple Heater Meridian becomes *kyo*, the skin and mucous membranes become oversensitive and manifest allergic reactions. Asthma may be caused by Lung *kyo*, but if it is caused by Triple Heater *kyo*, it is due to allergy. The typical conditions that cause colds are Triple Heater *jitsu*, which causes fevers, and Large Intestine *kyo*, which causes sore throat and a runny nose. Fever promotes peripheral circulation; therefore, what causes headaches with colds is the hardening of the *jitsu* in the Triple Heater Meridian in the head area. Triple Heater *jitsu*, caused by entering and leaving air-conditioned rooms and buildings, becomes more prevalent during the summer. Because the Triple Heater is responsible for adaptation to the outside world, going from a cold environment to a warm one overactivates this meridian.

One of my own patients had been diagnosed by an ear-nose-throat specialist as suffering from inflammation of the mucous membrane of the nose. According to this patient, she had been treated by the specialist for five years without result. On diagnosis I found that her nasal mucous membrane was oversensitive because her condition was Triple Heater *kyo*. I supplemented the *kyo* condition and she was cured within two months.

Liver and Gall Bladder

Statistically, there are fewer people with Gall Bladder *kyo* than there are with Liver *kyo*. However, when the *kyo* condition of the Gall Bladder worsens, it often turns into Liver *kyo*. One characteristic of Liver *kyo* is the tendency to become tired. Also, because the Gall Bladder and Liver Meridians control the muscles and joints in the whole body, Liver *kyo* weakens physical strength. Because the Gall Bladder Meridian controls secretion of the digestive juices, the *kyo* pattern of this meridian often manifests gastric imbalance, indicated by poor digestion of fats, obesity, and a feeling of nausea after eating.

The Classics note that disorders in the Liver and Gall Bladder Meridians are caused by diet. This is because these meridians are responsible for antidotal activity. (In ancient China, where meridians were said to function like a government, the Liver and Gall Bladder were likened to an army protecting the country from external attack.) In fact, *kyo* patterns of the Liver and Gall Bladder are often caused by consumption of products such as white sugar, alcohol, and foods that have chemical additives. These food toxins exacerbate the *kyo* condition and may also generate nervous disorders. One of my patients, a woman in her late twenties who exhibited intercostal muscle pain, revealed extreme Gall Bladder *kyo*, which had caused contraction and pain in the chest muscles. I wondered if it had anything to do with her diet and asked if she had been eating instant or sweet foods. She answered that she was especially fond of cakes, which she ate more than three times a day. Apart from white sugar, cakes contain preservatives and other additives. Treatment of disorders in patients who eat such foods daily often takes a long time, and unless the patient's dietary habits change, the disorder returns. I told this patient that her problem was caused by her diet and that she would not improve unless she stopped eating cakes. I asked her not to return for treatment until she had decided to change her diet. Some time later she contacted me to say she was ready to begin therapy. I then treated her twice weekly for three months, and her condition improved.

Conception Vessel and Governor Vessel

In the Classics, it is noted that the Conception and Governor Vessels play the role of bypass when there is poor circulation in the twelve meridians in the arms and legs. In the disciplines of *sendo*, practiced to heighten one's vital forces, these two meridians are of utmost importance (chapter 1). However, in ancient diagrams of meridians and in the diagrams of the twelve meridians throughout the body, the Conception and Governor Vessels are shown as running only on the back and front areas of the body, which meant there was no appropriate method of treating the *kyo-jitsu* conditions. But since the discovery of the twenty-four meridians throughout the body and the meridians that run along the sides of the body, it has become possible to perform effective treatment of these conditions by using the Governor and Conception Vessels in the limbs and back region.

In recent times, I have noticed an unexpected increase in the number of patients with the *kyo* pattern of the Conception and Governor Vessels, which, like the increase in Lung *kyo*, may be a manifestation of modern lifestyles. Although there are no particularly noticeable characteristic symptoms that arise from this pattern, patients with this condition may suffer from hemorrhoids, debility, or fatigue. Some may also complain of dizziness or shoulder stiffness and neck pain.

The Twenty-Four Meridians throughout the Body

The following pages present diagrams of the twenty-four meridians that flow throughout the body. The bold lines show the main meridians (the meridians indicated by Masunaga in his diagrams of the twelve meridians throughout the body) and the dotted lines show the sub-meridians. Solid dots indicate the last points of main meridians, while open dots indicate the last points of sub-meridians. Shaded regions are the areas occupied by the meridians in the *hara* or back.

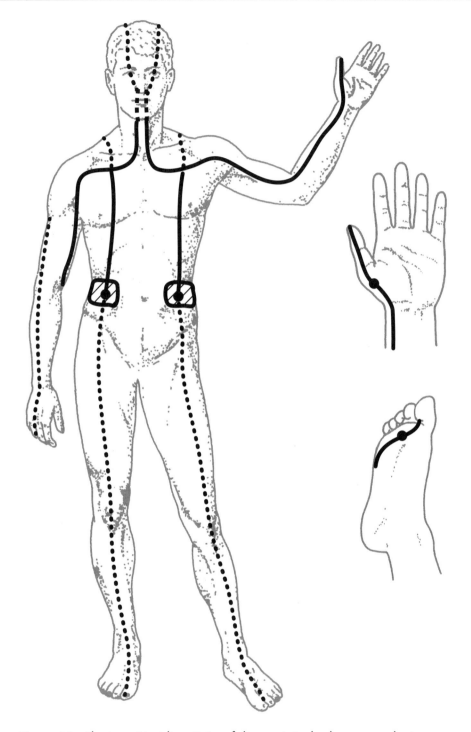

Figure 4.1 The Lung Meridian. Point of diagnosis in the *hara* area: the intersection of the horizontal line crossing the navel and the line joining the sternum and the anterior superior iliaca spina (ASIS).

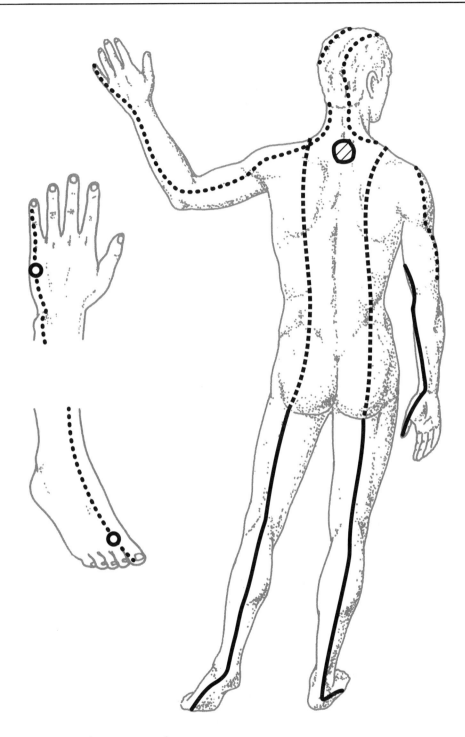

Figure 4.2   The Lung Meridian

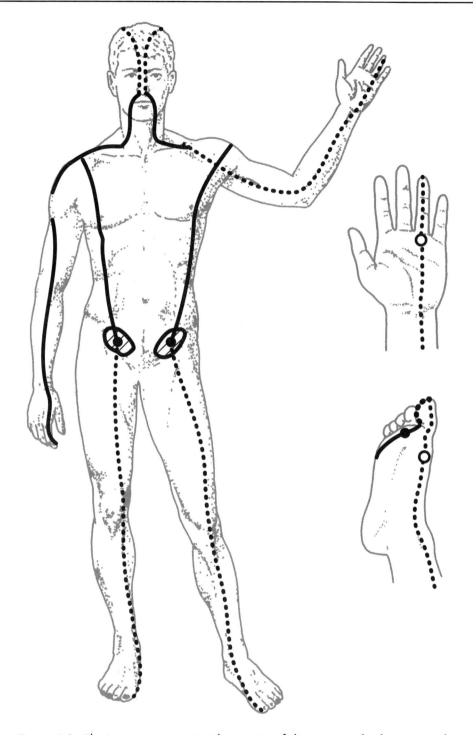

Figure 4.3 The Large Intestine Meridian. Point of diagnosis in the *hara* area: the midpoint of the line joining the pelvic bone and the ASIS.

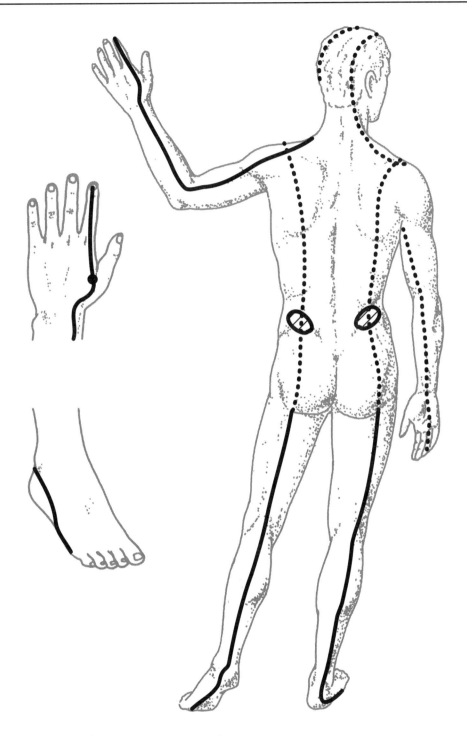

Figure 4.4   The Large Intestine Meridian

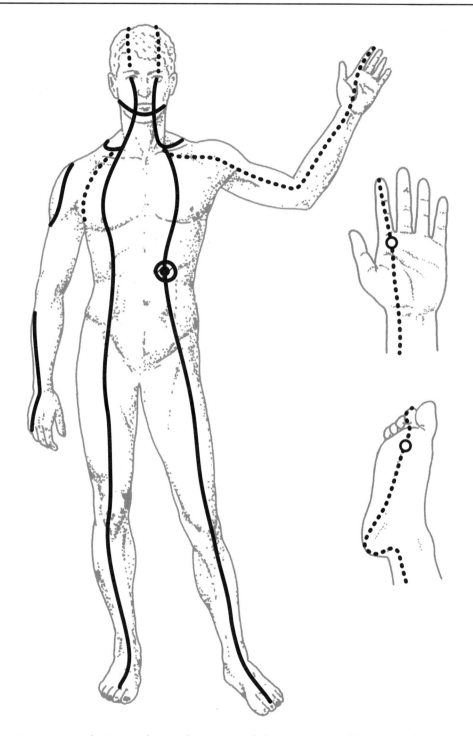

Figure 4.5 The Stomach Meridian. Point of diagnosis in the *hara* area: the intersection of the line from the End of Acromion to the ASIS and the horizontal line crossing the point of diagnosis of the Heart Meridian.

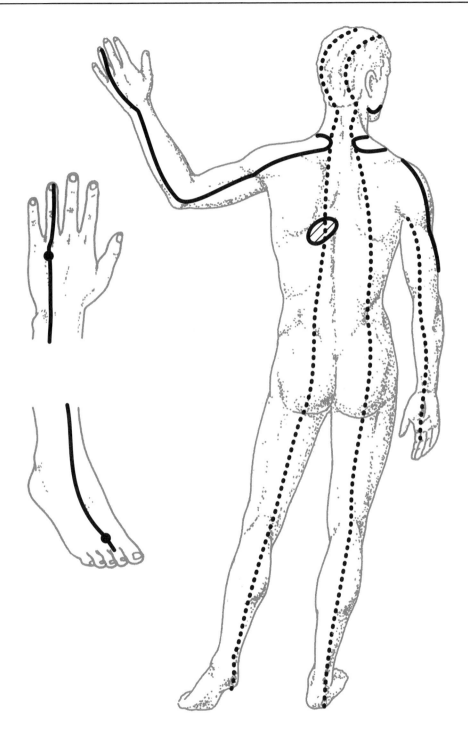

Figure 4.6   The Stomach Meridian

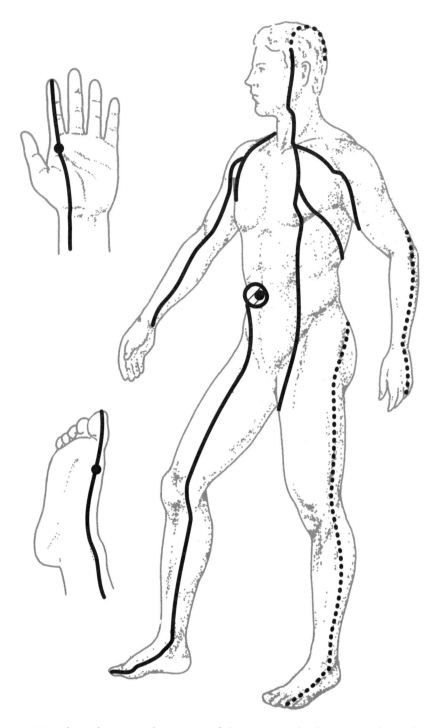

Figure 4.7   The Spleen Meridian. Point of diagnosis in the *hara* area: the mid-point of the line joining the navel and the point of diagnosis of the Heart constrictor.

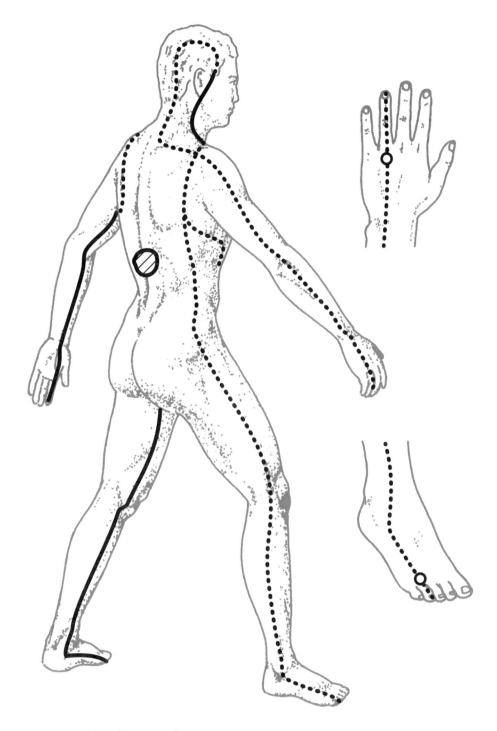

Figure 4.8   The Spleen Meridian

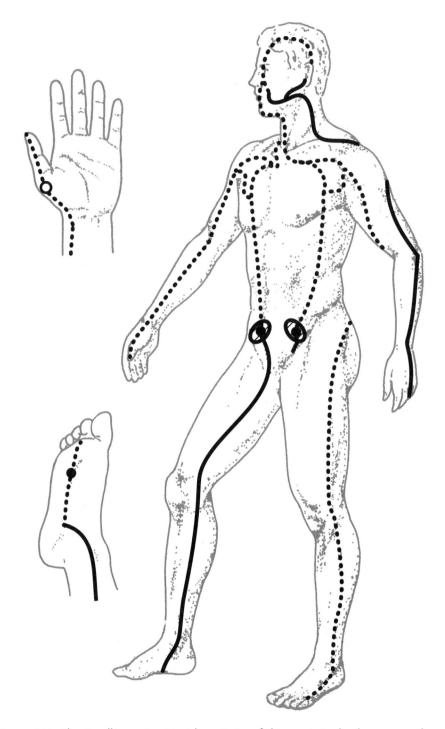

Figure 4.9 The Small Intestine Meridian. Point of diagnosis in the *hara* area: the intersection of the line joining the navel and the point of diagnosis of the Large Intestine Meridian and the horizontal line crossing the point of diagnosis of the Governor Vessel.

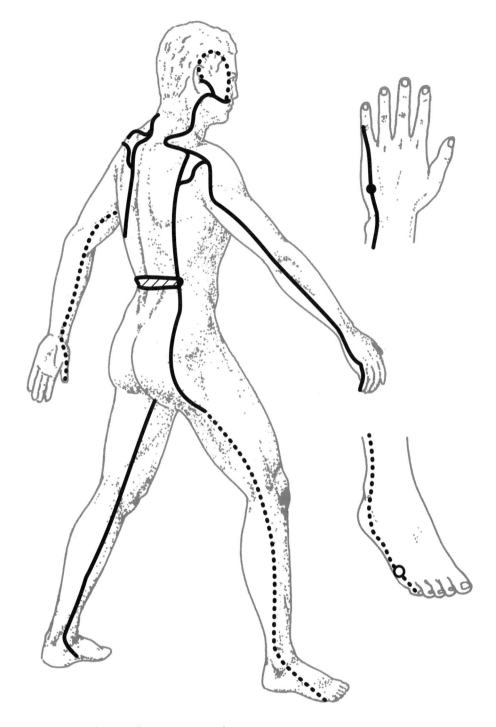

Figure 4.10   The Small Intestine Meridian

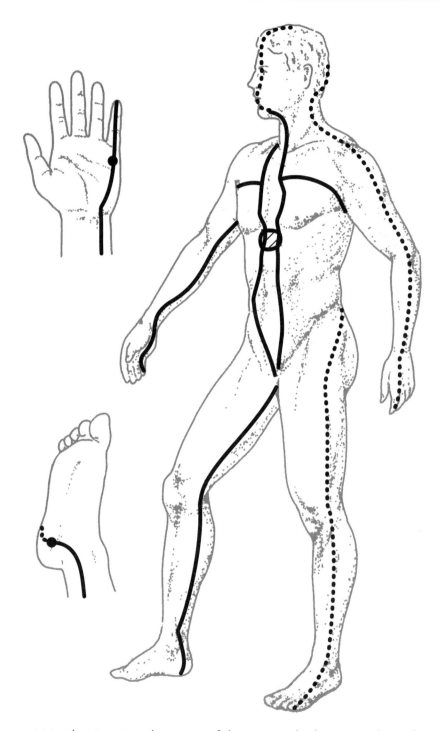

Figure 4.11   The Heart Meridian. Point of diagnosis in the *hara* area: the midpoint of the line joining the sternum and the point of diagnosis of the Heart Constrictor.

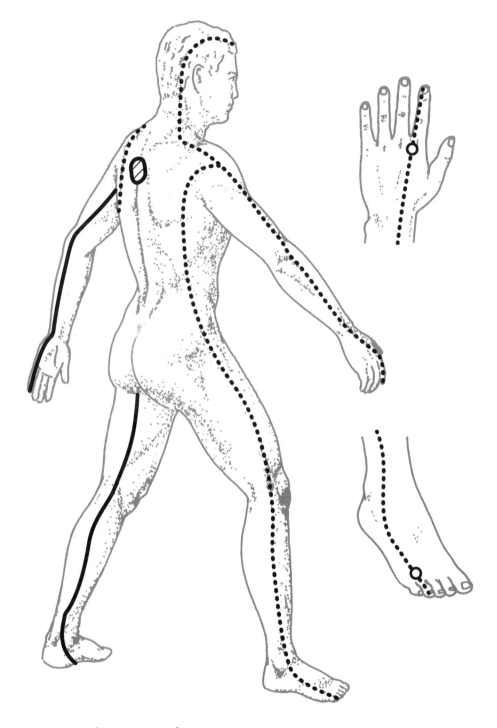

Figure 4.12   The Heart Meridian

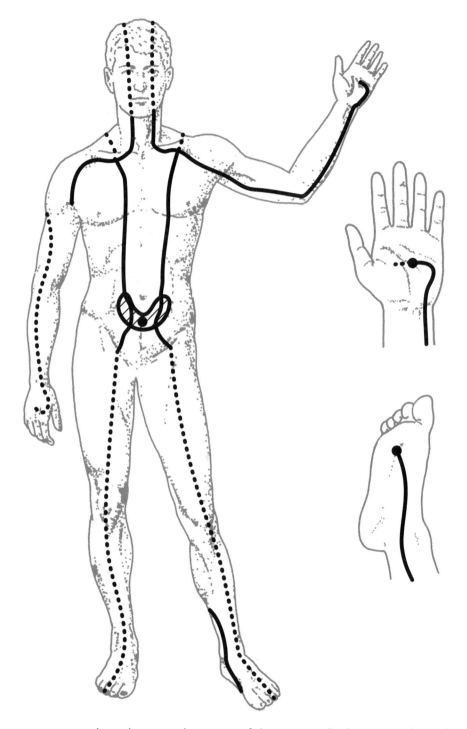

Figure 4.13 The Kidney Meridian. Point of diagnosis in the *hara* area: the midpoint of the line joining the pubic bone and the navel.

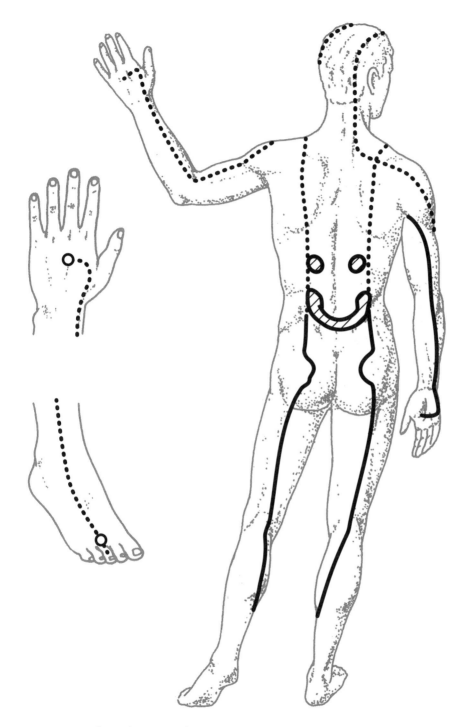

Figure 4.14 The Kidney Meridian

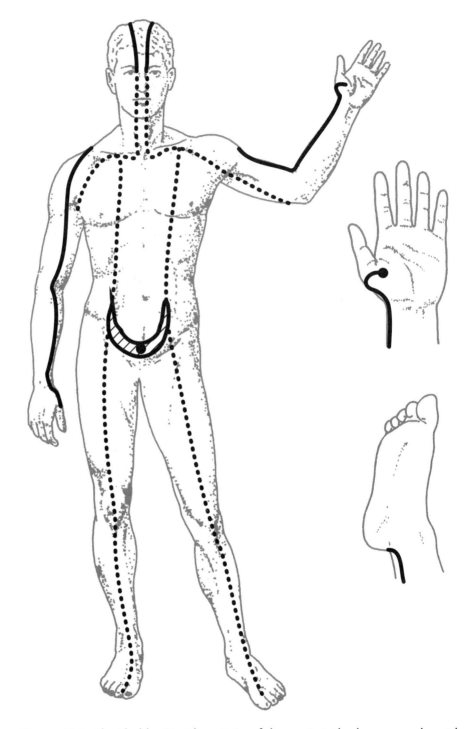

Figure 4.15 The Bladder Meridian. Point of diagnosis in the *hara* area: the midpoint of the line joining the point of diagnosis of the Kidney Meridian and the pubic bone.

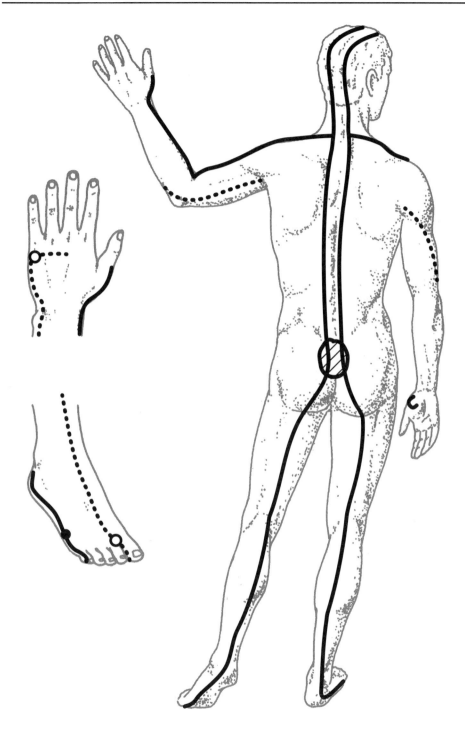

Figure 4.16   The Bladder Meridian

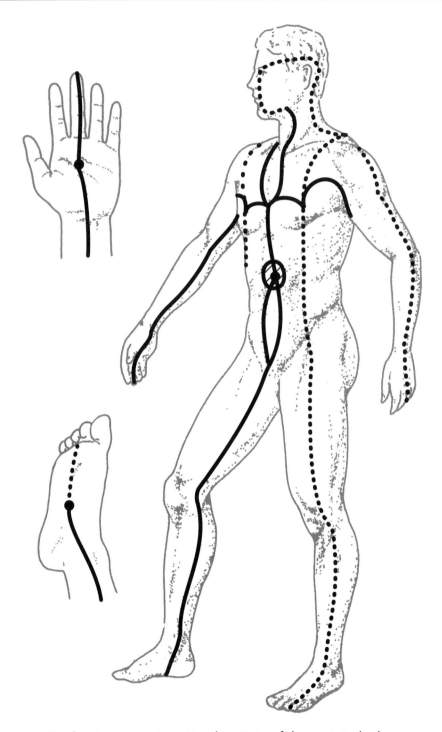

Figure 4.17 The Heart Constrictor Meridian. Point of diagnosis in the *hara* area: the midpoint of the line joining the navel and the sternum.

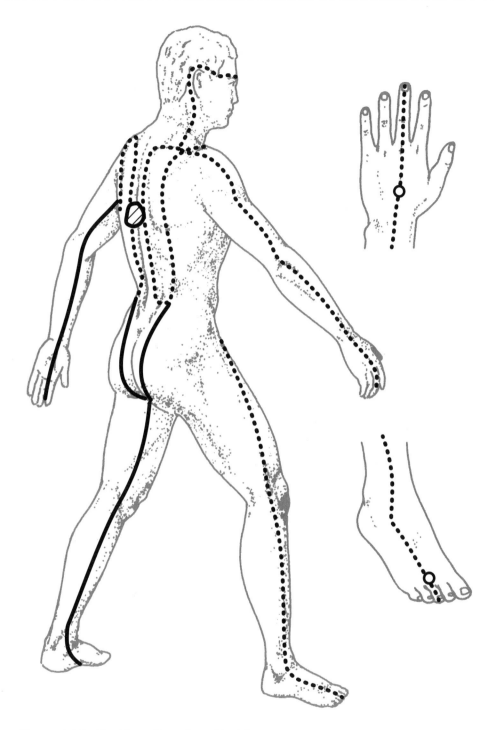

Figure 4.18   The Heart Constrictor Meridian

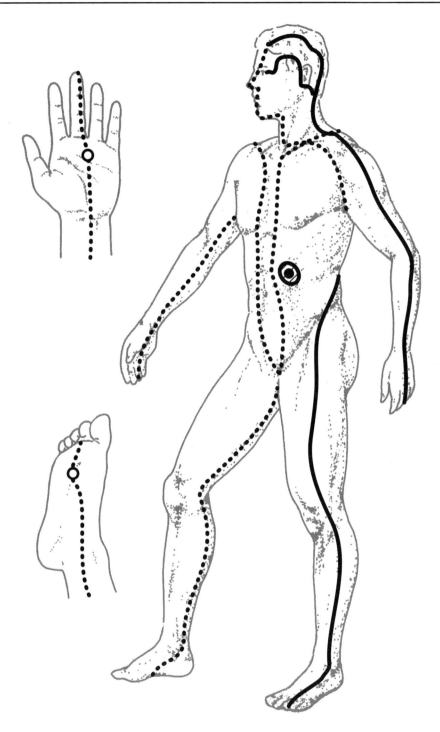

Figure 4.19 The Triple Heater Meridian. Point of diagnosis in the *hara* area: the intersection of the line joining the end of the acromion and the point of diagnosis of the Lung Meridian and the horizontal line crossing the point of diagnosis of the Spleen Meridian.

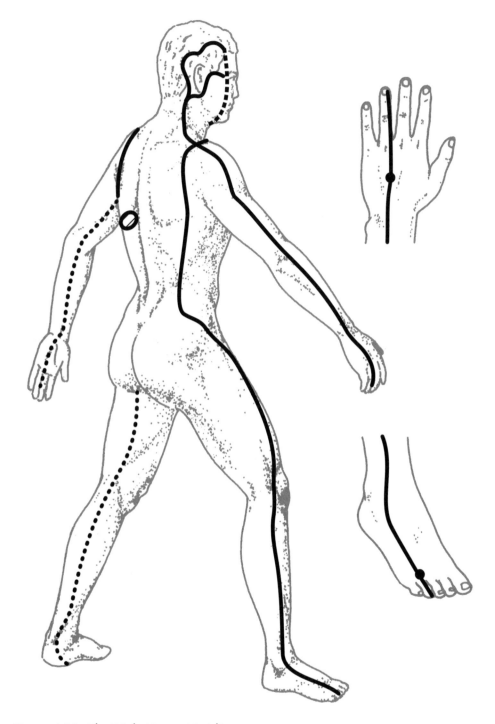

Figure 4.20   The Triple Heater Meridian

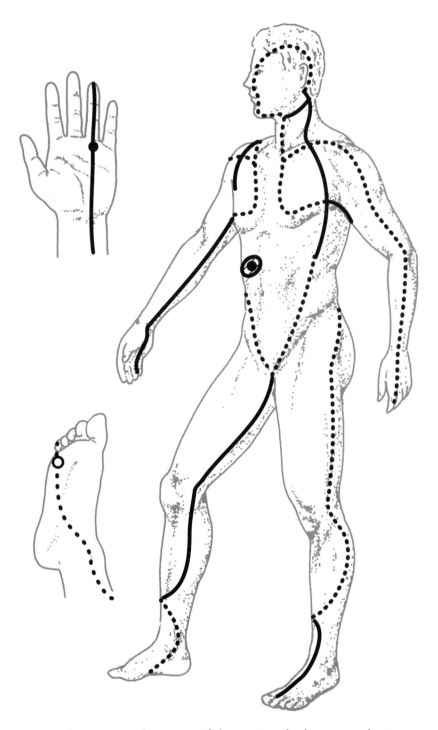

Figure 4.21   The Liver Meridian. Point of diagnosis in the *hara* area: the intersection of the line joining the sternum and the ASIS and the horizontal line from the midpoint between the points of diagnosis of the Heart Constrictor Meridian and the Spleen Meridian.

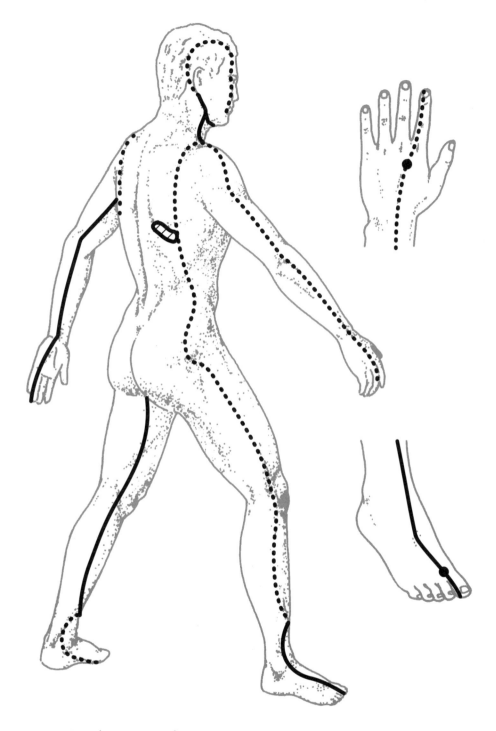

Figure 4.22   The Liver Meridian

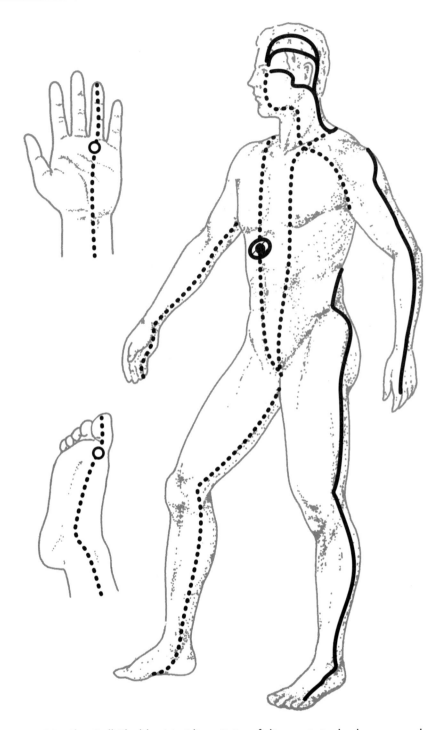

Figure 4.23 The Gall Bladder Meridian. Point of diagnosis in the *hara* area: the intersection of the line joining the ASIS and the point of diagnosis of the Heart Meridian and the horizontal line from the point of diagnosis of the Conception Vessel.

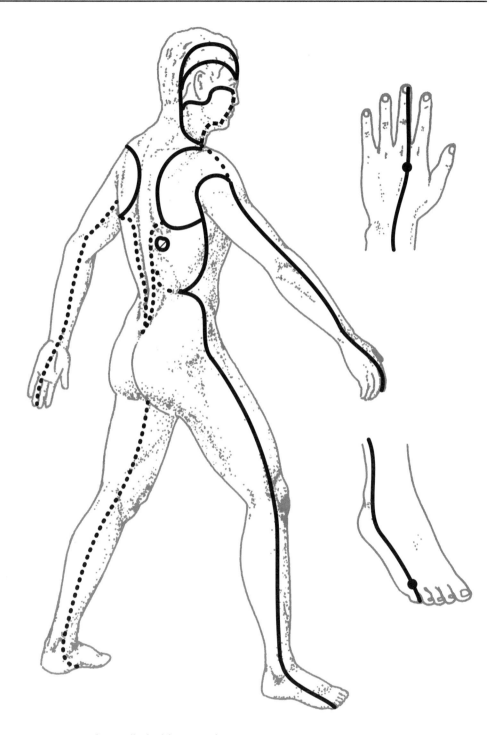

Figure 4.24   The Gall Bladder Meridian

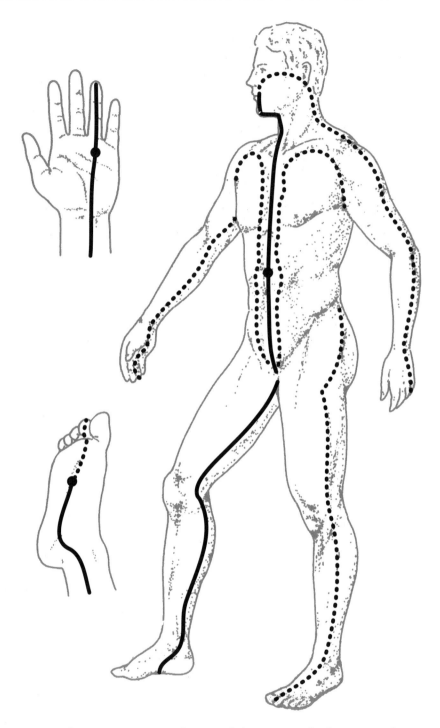

Figure 4.25 The Conception Vessel. Point of diagnosis in the *hara* area: the midpoint of the line joining the point of diagnosis of the Heart Constrictor and the navel.

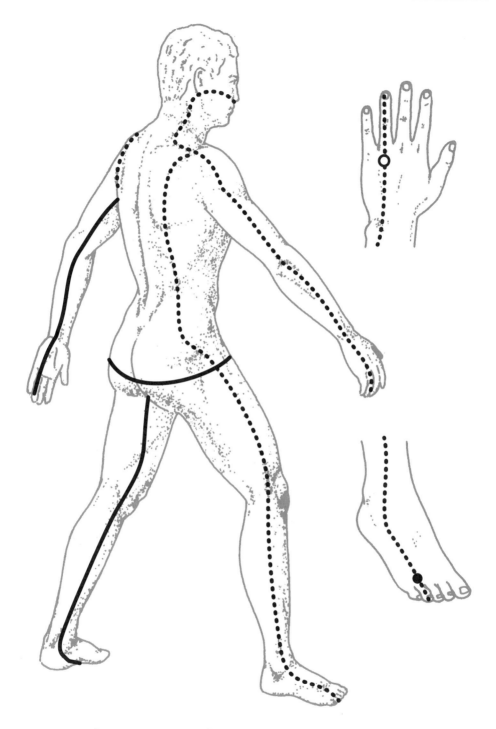

Figure 4.26   The Conception Vessel

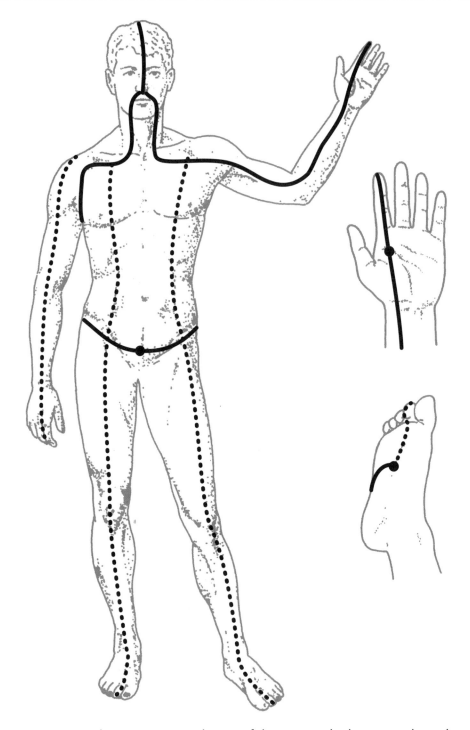

Figure 4.27 The Governor Vessel. Point of diagnosis in the *hara* area: the midpoint of the line joining the point of diagnosis of the Kidney Meridian and the point of diagnosis of the Bladder Meridian.

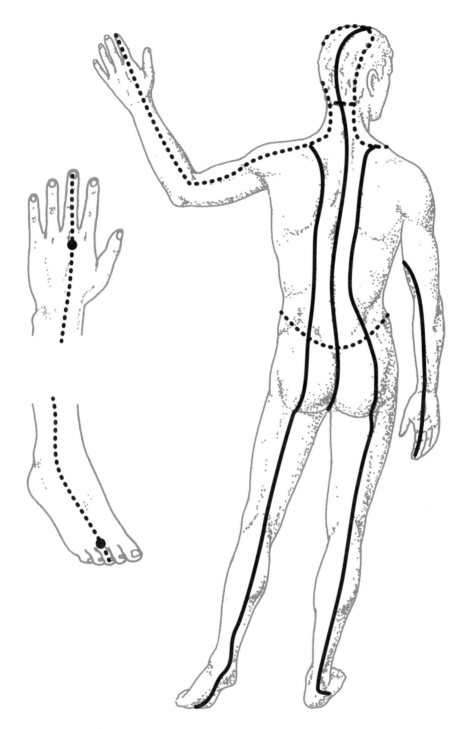

Figure 4.28   The Governor Vessel

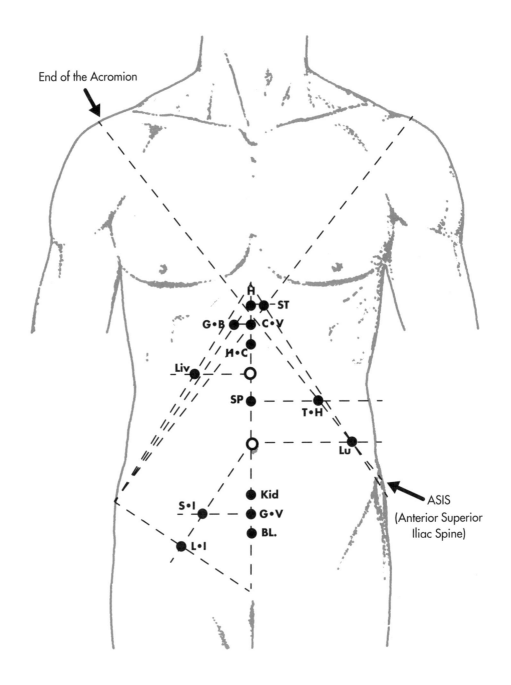

Figure 4.29 Points of Diagnosis in the *Hara* Area

Chapter Five

Meridianal Therapy

Tsubo and Meridians

Definition of *Tsubo*

Physiological Depressions on the Meridians.   Generally, *tsubo* are called acupuncture points; however, the *tsubo* used in Tao shiatsu are not considered to be as anatomically positioned. A *tsubo* is considered to be a physiological depression that changes according to particular circumstances. Meridianal therapy cannot be performed without the access provided by the *tsubo*, which play an extremely important role in treating the *kyo* meridians. The *kyo* meridians not only run along the surface of the body but also lie deep within the body. *Tsubo* are the points of therapy appearing above the meridians, and the *kyo* meridians cannot be perceived without actually touching these points. (See Figure 5.1.) Without an understanding of *tsubo*, meridians can only be recognized as lines running along the surface of the body and not as phenomena of life. We do not know why such physiological depressions are manifested on the meridians. However, because they appear as depressions, they are perceived as "holes." *Tsubo* are the windows or doors through which the meridians are reached. Therefore, more than simple physiological depressions, they are important points for treatment.

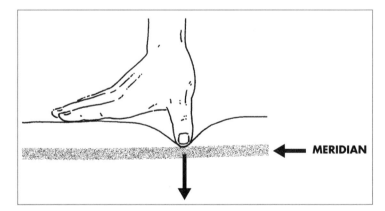

Figure 5.1

Points on Which the Patient Subconsciously Requires Shiatsu. The healer decides which *tsubo* to treat by observing the patient's whole body and determining the points where shiatsu pressure is most required. Students often ask if the *tsubo* are found by touching the patient's body, but the sense of touch can only perceive one part of the body at a time, which is contrary to the holistic nature of Oriental medicine. Shiatsu does not rely on the sense of touch but is performed through a heightened primal sense that first examines the patient holistically and, second, recognizes where the pressure is most needed. Therefore, the healer must begin with visual diagnosis that reveals the different depth of each *tsubo*. Then, through a heightened primal sense, the healer takes the most deeply positioned *tsubo* as the points of therapy.

Because *tsubo*, like meridians, do not actually exist within the physical body, their depth is not easily determined through accepted standards of known measurements. Both *tsubo* and meridians belong in the realm of the body of *ki;* therefore, the true depth of a *tsubo* lies beyond the physical body and may be from around one and a half to around three meters from the surface of the skin. Selecting a *tsubo* as the point where the patient requires shiatsu means that the healer must understand its true depth as a three-dimensional position rather than a position along the surface of the body. For instance, if the true depth of the *tsubo* is determined to be two meters, the healer must visualize this because only through visualization can the healer's *ki* reach that depth.

Points that Affect the Whole Body. *Tsubo* are points of depression deficient in *ki*. Therefore, when constant steady pressure is applied, they fill with *ki* and disappear from that particular area of the body (see Figure 5.2). However, if shiatsu continues even after a *tsubo* has filled with *ki* and disappeared, the patient begins to resist the pressure and feel pain. At this point, the meridians sustain some damage, causing the symptoms to deteriorate. Discontinuation of pressure is determined by the depth of the particular *tsubo* being treated, and the healer's degree of pressure and skill. For instance, as the *tsubo* fills with *ki*, the skilled healer senses when the patient is satisfied and the depression resolved.

To locate a *tsubo* on, for instance, the forearm, the healer observes the entire forearm and looks for the point that most requires shiatsu. These are the points that produce an effect on the rest of the forearm, produce an echo in

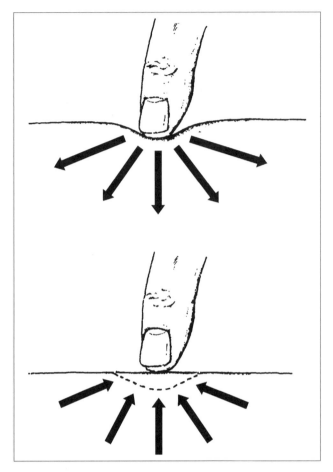

Figure 5.2

another part of the arm (a sensation that the other part is also being pressed), and affect the whole arm.

The Points of Contact of the *Kyo* Meridians. The *kyo* meridians, apart from those indicated in most meridianal diagrams, include those that run horizontally throughout the body and the Spiral Meridian (see Figure 5.3). A *tsubo* is the depression formed at the point of contact of the horizontal meridians with the *kyo* meridians. Sometimes a reaction to *tsubo* treatment is felt in areas of the body that do not correspond to the lines on meridianal diagrams. This is because the response is occurring in the Spiral Meridian and the horizontal meridians, which are not yet indicated in such diagrams.

Three Rules of *Tsubo* Therapy

1. Visualizing the Cushion of *Ki.* Although there are some principles common to both basic shiatsu and meridianal *tsubo* therapy, there are also definite differences. One fundamental difference is that in basic shiatsu, the skin is moved by taking up the slack of the skin (chapter 2), whereas in *tsubo* therapy, pressure is applied to the surface of the body in a perpendicular direction.

The *tsubo* on the *kyo* meridians are generally soft and weak on the surface but hard underneath. The *kyo* induration, which may be likened to a toxic mass (or energy block) caused by stagnant or deficient *ki*, exists deep within the *tsubo.* When this is treated with therapeutic *ki*, it gradually dissolves and the related illness is healed. It must be remembered that although the *tsubo* at the mouth of the *kyo* induration is the point of healing, it is also a point of

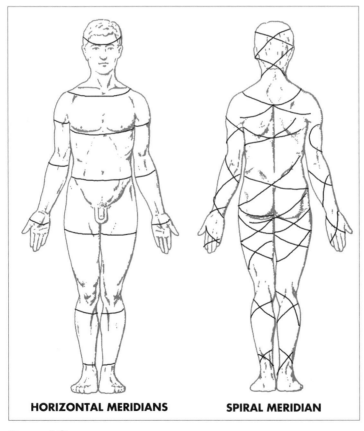

HORIZONTAL MERIDIANS   **SPIRAL MERIDIAN**

Figure 5.3

weakness that may be damaged when touched directly, causing injury to the patient's meridians. Therefore, the shiatsu techniques of visualization (chapter 1) are necessary for *tsubo* therapy. Rather than applying pressure directly, as though to reach the bottom of the *tsubo* with the fingers, the healer must maintain the pressure while visualizing a cushion of *ki* two or three millimeters thick between the fingers and the patient's body (see Figures 5.4 and 5.5). Furthermore, the shiatsu healers should also visualize a "bubble" in the *ki* cushion (see Figure 5.6). This *ki* bubble actually exists at a depth of 1.5 millimeters and the healer must visualize applying pressure to it rather than to the physical body so as not to cause damage to the patient.

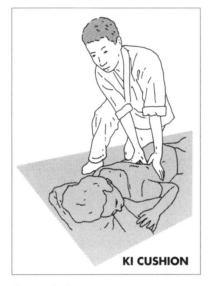

KI CUSHION

KI CUSHION

Figure 5.4

Figure 5.5

To avoid possible meridianal damage from direct physical touch, the healer must maintain this image throughout the application of pressure. This means that *ki*, and not the healer's fingers, is directing the pressure. If the image is interrupted for any reason, the healer should stop applying pressure on that *tsubo*. This technique is not an easy one to follow: if the pressure is too shallow, the effect will be weak, and if the image of the cushion of *ki* is not strong enough, the meridian will be damaged. The correct degree of pressure is that which makes the pressure felt throughout the patient's body.

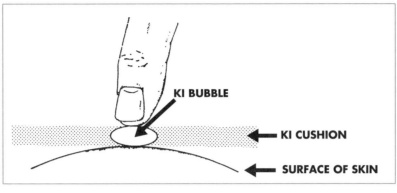

Figure 5.6

One method of determining whether the *tsubo* treatment is effective is to observe the depth of the patient's breath. When continuous pressure is applied to a *tsubo*, if it is effective, the patient's breath deepens. If, however, the breath becomes more shallow, even if the patient feels no pain, the pressure is probably inappropriate and may lead to some degree of meridianal damage.

2. Unification of the Points of Contact with the Patient and the Earth.   In addition to visualizing the cushion of *ki*, one must also maintain an image of the oneness of the fingers (the points of contact with the patient) and the knees and tips of the toes (the points of contact with the earth). To determine whether this image is being maintained, use the simple test described in chapter 2. Healers who maintain the image effectively do not fall when pushed from the side during therapy, nor can their feet be lifted from the floor.

3. Equalizing the Action and Reaction. The action is the degree of pressure the patient receives and the reaction is the patient's response to that pressure. These two must be perfectly balanced: if the healer focuses only on the applied pressure, the pressure becomes too severe for the patient. Therefore, the pressure must be constant and the healer must always be aware of the balance between the pressure and the patient's response. The patient's response to pressure flows from the Conception Vessel in the healer's arms to the *tanden* and the Governor Vessel in the healer's legs, and through to the center of the earth. When appropriate pressure is applied, the action and reaction are perfectly balanced.

Order of *Tsubo* Therapy

Tsubo treatment should always be carried out in the following order:

1. Observing the Whole Body. Before actually touching the patient, the healer must first of all observe the patient's whole body in order to ascertain where he or she requires pressure.

As explained earlier, the sense of touch is inadequate for searching for a *tsubo*, because the patient's *ki* must be sensed through the primal sense. Therefore the healer must always search for the *tsubo* by visual observation.

2. Determining the Position of the *Tsubo* through Index Finger Pressure. To ascertain the *tsubo* through pressure of the index finger, the healer should touch the surface of the patient's skin very lightly. This allows the healer's *ki* to reach the true depth of the patient's *tsubo* (about one and a half to three meters below the surface of the skin). Actually applying pressure with the fingers enables the healer's *ki* to sympathize with the patient's true *tsubo*.

3. Actual Application of Pressure. The healer does not actually apply pressure or touch the patient's body until after visualizing the cushion of *ki*. When the pressure has reached the appropriate depth, the healer asks the patient the following questions:

"How does it feel?" Effective shiatsu may, for example, feel good even though it is painful, while uncomfortable shiatsu may result in damage. Therefore, this question must be asked first.

"Does it echo?" The echo is a sensation that the pressure is reaching areas not actually being pressed. The echo can be sensed in other parts of the body where there is pain or numbness. However, when *kyo* is chronic and deep, the echo can be felt deep within the *tsubo* being pressed. The patient does not always necessarily feel an echo, but usually, if correct *tsubo* shiatsu pressure is being applied, the patient will feel one. When the patient does not feel an echo, the healer should ask the patient whether the depth and angle of the pressure on that particular *tsubo* feel appropriate.

"Has the pressure lasted long enough?" There is no fixed period of time for the application of pressure on a particular *tsubo*. However, when the *tsubo* has filled with *ki*, patients sense that they have had enough and are able to convey this to the healer. When the *tsubo* has filled with *ki*, the degree of pressure (that is, the depth of pressure) should be weakened gradually.

It is important to remember that to ensure that the therapy is truly effective, the healer must always ask the patient these questions. The healer must *never* feel completely self-assured that the therapy is correct and must *always* be cautious not to damage the patient's body of *ki*. In addition, the ideal pressure for the *tsubo* is changing from moment to moment. The *tsubo* is trying to rise to the surface in reaction to the therapist's *ki*. Therefore, the therapist must keep adapting the level of pressure to suit the depth of the *tsubo* at each moment.

The Practice of Meridianal Therapy

As a rule in shiatsu, *sho* diagnosis and meridianal therapy are not performed until after performing the basic techniques on patients lying on their side and face down. This is because *sho* diagnosis taken after basic shiatsu reveals deeper disorders and enables more effective meridianal therapy.

Meridianal therapy may be broadly divided between the arms and legs, the symptoms, and the *hara*. Among these, the order of therapy is determined purely according to each individual patient. Whatever form of meridianal therapy is chosen, the basic rule is always to apply shiatsu on the *tsubo* pertaining to the meridians where the patient exhibits a response. If the *kyo* of the main meridians is very deep, it is necessary to treat the sub-meridians on the opposite side of the body first. For instance, because *kyo* in the *hara* area is generally quite deep, treatment is first of all carried out on the lower back area. Similarly, the *kyo* pattern in the back region is first treated with shiatsu on the chest.

Meridianal Therapy on the Arms and Legs

The basic method of meridianal therapy on the arms and legs is carried out on the deepest *tsubo* of the meridians, directing the pressure toward the extremities of the limbs. It must be remembered that when the *kyo* in the main meridians is overly deep, therapy is first performed on the sub-meridians and then on the main meridians. However, there are times when therapy should be performed on the sub-meridians in the thighs and times when it should be performed on the main meridians in the lower legs. The healer should try both methods to see which is more effective. In each case, applying continuous pressure to the extremities of the sub-meridians on which diagnosis and therapy are being performed is very effective. When performing meridianal therapy on the arms and legs, after diagnosis of the *kyo-jitsu* pattern, the healer should begin therapy on the *kyo* side, followed by the *jitsu* side. See Figure 5.7 for some points on the meridians in the arms and legs.

Since the *kyo-jitsu* pattern indicates the balance of yin and yang, it may be manifested throughout the body, in the meridians, or on the left or right side of the body. The side of the body that uses most energy and is the strongest is *jitsu*, and the other side is *kyo*. For instance, if one is right-handed, the right arm is generally *jitsu*. The foot one tends to put out first when walking is also

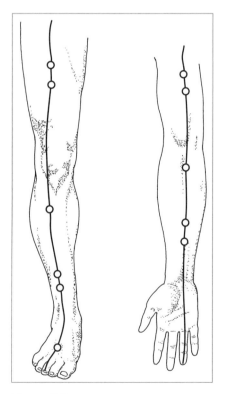

Figure 5.7

usually *jitsu*. The side of the body most prone to injury is usually the *jitsu* side, because in accidents, people unconsciously protect their *kyo* side. When the *kyo* side is injured, the injury not only is more serious but also takes longer to heal than a similar one on the *jitsu* side. When the *jitsu* side of the body is bruised, the bruising disappears when shiatsu is applied immediately to the *kyo* meridians on the *kyo* side. However, this is not the case with bruises on the *kyo* side. Because *kyo* is a weakness, a strike with the same force causes more damage to the *kyo* side than to the *jitsu* side.

See Figures 5.8 and 5.9 for an explanation of *sho* diagnosis on the right and left sides of the body. In the legs (Figure 5.8), the side that extends freely, without force, is *kyo*. In the arms (Figure 5.9), the side that sits more firmly on the floor is *jitsu*.

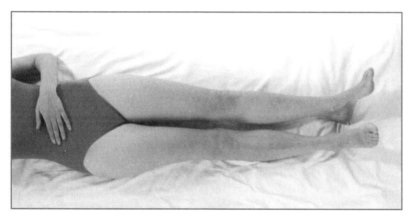

Figure 5.8

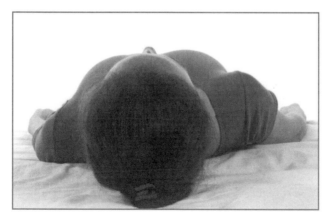

Figure 5.9

Symptoms and Meridianal Therapy

The symptoms discussed here are physical discomforts such as back pain and neck or shoulder stiffness. Other symptoms, such as coughing, palpitations, headache, or fever, may be cured by the basic shiatsu techniques and meridianal therapy to the *hara*, legs, and arms. (The details of shiatsu therapy for other symptoms are explained in detail in Masunaga's *Zen Shiatsu.*[1]) There is an infinite variety of pain symptoms of similar ailments and tension that occur when the patient moves, remains still, or both. Furthermore, a stiffness, whether it be *jitsu, kyo,* or a mixture of both, can be equally painful whether it is deep or forms lumps on the surface of the body.

Pain and stiffness are not always specific. It is well known that diseases of the internal organs can generate uncomfortable stiffness in the back or other areas of the body. This is caused by a reaction in the lining or wall of the affected organs. Shiatsu therapy directed at tension in the wall of such organs can cure the disease. By healing tension deep in the internal organs that has not yet become obvious on the surface, it is possible to cure an illness before it manifests any symptoms.

Since treatment differs according to the symptoms, one must diagnose the symptoms as either *kyo* or *jitsu* before beginning treatment. Therefore, the healer must be familiar with the characteristics of *kyo* and *jitsu* in order to diagnose the symptoms. To begin with, *kyo* symptoms are manifested deep within the body and not on the surface, and because these are characteristically yin, they belong in the realm of the subconscious rather than that of the conscious. It is difficult to conceptualize the deeper parts of the body, so characteristic *kyo* symptoms are not easily recognized by the amateur. *Kyo* discomfort is felt deep inside the body rather than in individual parts, and patients are often not able to accurately identify which part of their body is hurting.

Jitsu symptoms, on the other hand, exhibit superficial pain. These can be relatively easily identified by the patient, and because they harden on the surface, even the amateur healer can feel their presence (see Figure 5.10). *Jitsu* symptoms can be comparatively easily treated by finding and treating the *kyo* meridian. *Jitsu* symptoms may improve through basic whole-body shiatsu and *sha* therapy on the *jitsu* meridian. Because *jitsu* is characteristically

---

1. Shizuto Masunaga, *Zen Shiatsu* (Tokyo: Japan Publications, 1977).

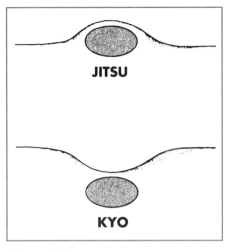

Figure 5.10

yang and a state of stagnation of energy, it has the strength to cure itself through appropriate stimulation. Effective treatment is readily available, since *jitsu* pain and stiffness can be relieved by direct use of acupuncture needles. However, the essence of therapy shows that, because *jitsu* is generated by *kyo*, the *jitsu* will continue to reappear as long as the *kyo* is not fulfilled. It is therefore inadequate to simply relieve the symptoms. This is why acupuncture needles are often used in conjunction with moxibustion. In other words, initially, in order to supplement the needles of the *sha* method (yang) on the *jitsu*, *ho* moxa cautery (yin) is used on the *kyo*. (Moxa cautery functions as *ho* because it feeds fire energy into the *kyo* meridians.) As can be seen from such therapeutic techniques, acupuncture and moxibustion have the yin-yang relationship.

Kyo symptoms require a more highly skilled technique and sense of sympathy than *jitsu* symptoms. For instance, treating the area of a *kyo* symptom caused by physical and psychological damage to the patient's *ki* with *sha* therapy may result in deterioration of the condition being treated. Because *kyo* is an injury generated in the body of *ki* (the ether body), the healer performing touch therapy must channel *ki* into it in order to heal the injury. However, treating *kyo* symptoms with *sha* therapy makes injury move even deeper. This is because rather than enhancing *ki*, the *sha* method reduces it. *Sha* therapy is rhythmical pressure applied by placing one hand on the area manifesting the symptoms and using the other hand to apply pressure on the meridian in the same part of the body for one second on each point (see Figure 5.11). This is repeated twice.

Generally, *jitsu* is acute and *kyo* is chronic, though chronic *jitsu* symptoms and acute *kyo* symptoms are also possible. When a pain that originally surfaced in the right leg is cured and moves to the left leg, an *acute jitsu* symptom (the pain in the right leg) has become *chronic kyo* (the pain in the left leg). Pain in the right leg does not indicate that the problem originated there; rather, in order to protect the *kyo* in the left leg, *jitsu* carries the burden of the disorder. When the disorder is minimal, it does not manifest *kyo* pain, but major disorders develop into deep *kyo*, which manifests severe discomfort and pain. In such cases, *jitsu* ceases to carry the burden of the disorder, and the pain moves from the right leg to the left. In other words, a part of the body that was not initially painful manifests symptoms of pain, indicating the existence of *kyo*, and even when the pain in the right leg is relieved, the disorder not has been cured.

There is an infinite variety of *kyo* symptoms and it is impossible to list all the techniques for their treatment. I believe that true shiatsu practice begins after the healer masters *sho* diagnosis, because the area of *kyo* stiffness or tension differs with each patient and true shiatsu therapy means being able to perform appropriate treatment on that area. (Where *jitsu* symptoms are

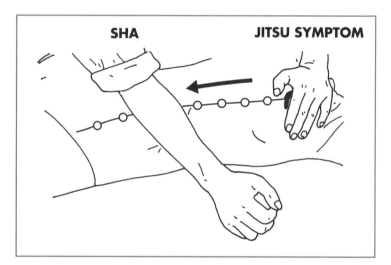

Figure 5.11

concerned, it is not necessary to locate the *kyo* tension because it is sufficient to simply supplement *kyo* after diagnosis.)

There are also symptoms that are a combination of both *kyo* and *jitsu*, which are manifested as *jitsu* in one area and *kyo* in another. In such cases the *jitsu* symptoms are treated first, and when these resolve, therapy is performed on the *kyo* symptoms. The simplest way of determining whether the symptoms are *kyo* or *jitsu* is to ask the patient whether the stiffness or pain is deep or superficial. But the healer cannot immediately assume that a deep discomfort is *kyo* and a superficial discomfort is *jitsu*, as there are cases where the patient complains of "deep pain" that turns out to be *jitsu*. The most reliable diagnostic method is to touch the surface of the painful area; if it is hard and tight, it is *jitsu*, and if it feels weak with a deep induration, it is *kyo*. The *jitsu* symptoms always appear after the *kyo* symptoms are resolved.

To treat symptoms, first of all place one hand on the pain or stiffness and move it as though to rock or shake the patient. Then ask the patient where he or she felt the most reaction. The part of the body that clearly manifests a response is the *tsubo* that evacuates toxins. This *tsubo* should be the point of therapy. These areas in which the points exist are fixed in the body, as shown in Figure 5.12. The *tsubo* at the extremities of the sub-meridians in the feet are also very effective in expelling toxins.

Meridianal Therapy on the *Hara* Region

Because the fundamental source of illness exists deep within the *kyo* induration in the *hara*, meridianal therapy on the *hara* region can be one of the most important methods of treatment. Remember that only through empathy can the healer discover the depth of the *kyo* induration. Treatment of a deep *kyo* induration is the basic method of restoring *ki* through empathy. The *kyo* meridians in the *hara* region are generally soft on the surface and hard underneath, and the basic method of meridianal treatment in this region is the *teate* technique used to warm the deep induration. Touching the *kyo* induration in the *hara* effectively heals disorders in parts of the body such as the back and lower back, and touch diagnosis may continue for as long as the response is favorable. Once this response stops, the disorder has been relieved. When the response is strong in an area of the patient's body other than the *hara*, the healer should place one hand on that area. The *kyo*

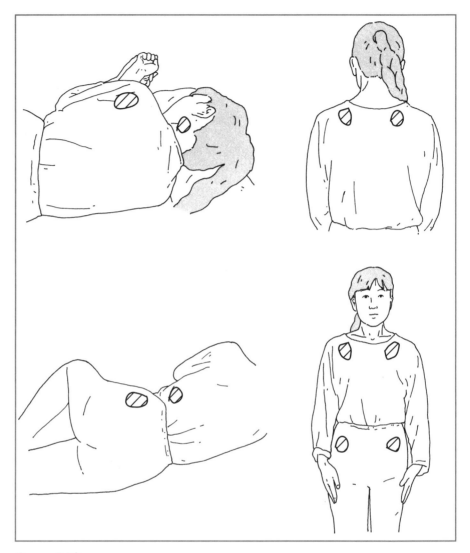

Figure 5.12

induration must never be struck carelessly or pressed forcefully. As it warms up, the healer, continuing to feel the patient's whole body, lifts his or her hand from the *hara* just enough to leave the thickness of one piece of paper between it and the patient. (Technically, this can be achieved by visualizing the cushion of *ki*.)

Even though maintaining the pressure on the patient's whole body as well as the space between the induration and the healer's hand may seem impossible to achieve, touch diagnosis cannot be performed without the integration of these two techniques. The *kyo* induration can only dissolve through the healer's ability to maintain this dual state, and in Tao shiatsu, therapy depends on whether the *kyo* induration in the *hara* region has been relieved.

However, this does not mean that it is sufficient to perform shiatsu only on the *hara* area. Whole-body therapy also relieves the *kyo* induration in the *hara* to some extent and shiatsu on the *hara* heightens the therapeutic result. In other words, the double effect of both whole-body shiatsu and *hara* shiatsu is the true result of therapy.

The Philosophy of Meridianal Therapy

Complying with the Patient's Vital Desires

Determining which *tsubo* are most in need of shiatsu therapy and applying pressure on them means complying with the patient's natural, vital requirements. For healers who try to determine the patient's vital demands and perform shiatsu therapy where the patient needs it, the world of *sho* of Oriental medicine is soon opened. In Chinese medicine, *sho* is expressed as *mei*, a word meaning clarity, discernment, wisdom. Just as we must have clarity in order to see matter, so too must we have an unclouded wisdom of the essence of life in order to discern *sho* and meridians. This wisdom (the *mei* of Chinese medicine) can be attained in shiatsu through compliance with the patient's vital desires, not through intellectualization.

As indicated by the visualization technique (chapter 1), correct understanding of meridians is not possible if shiatsu is studied and practiced as a merely mechanical or physical method. Those who understand shiatsu as a psychological technique and link the practice to their own spiritual advancement are able to touch the meridians, the profound existence of life. Meridians cannot be recognized by those who do not have the mentality to do so. Meridianal therapy is an intensely spiritual act and meridians can only begin to be recognized through selfless empathy toward the patient's life. Therefore, I believe that healers must perform shiatsu on the *tsubo* earnestly, from the bottom of their heart. This earnestness is not limited to shiatsu but is also common to other spiritual disciplines. Zen, for instance, preaches that one must "meditate earnestly" without desiring enlightenment. Buddhism also preaches earnest concentration on repetition of the sutras.

Indeed, such earnest concentration applies to other aspects of life also. If one hopes for success, it is important to act earnestly without selfish desires for personal advantages. This is because earnestness is born of the mental attitude that embraces the joys of others as one's own. Even where success is achieved, if it is exclusively to the individual's advantage without consideration of others, it is only temporary and utterly different from true success. This is because the laws of life are such that one cannot exist independently of other lives in the "whole." When we give pleasure to others, the pleasure is returned to us as a natural response from universal life.

In order to comply with the demands of the patient's life-force, it is necessary to empathetically understand the *ki* unconsciously desired by the patient and to perform shiatsu on the *tsubo* and meridians based on this empathy. As such, treating the *tsubo* is not a question of where the pressure is needed but rather what type of pressure is most appropriate. When a healer with a mind in empathy with the patient's needs presses a *tsubo*, the result is completely different from that of an action that seems to be exactly the same but is performed by a healer with a strong conscious sense of the self. This is because shiatsu performed with empathy releases *ki* in the body and creates therapeutically advantageous results, whereas shiatsu performed forcefully (with a strong sense of self) causes the body to become defensive, generating therapeutically disadvantageous results. Furthermore, since *tsubo* are located in vulnerable areas that cannot be protected by the body, inappropriate shiatsu may cause damage.

Illness exists because of mental, physical, and social restrictions. Relieving illness in order to restore freedom means empathizing with patients who live within such restrictions. The Western psychologist Carl Rogers emphasized the therapeutic effect of such sympathy and counseled patients by listening closely to what they said without psychoanalyzing them. This treatment is effective not only for neurosis but also for schizophrenia, and it has become the basis of a broad range of psychotherapies.

Because it embraces the natural healing powers within the patient's own body, counseling is also common to the methods of Oriental medicine, and in its empathy with the patient, counseling closely resembles shiatsu therapy. What counseling and shiatsu therapy have in common is that neither tries to correct or change the patient and that through empathy, the patient's suppressed energy is catalyzed, liberating the body and mind. Meridianal therapy requires a close familiarity with the common aspects of shiatsu and psychotherapy, because *tsubo* are not only the points of therapy but also the source of disorders in the patient's mind and body and are closely related to the patient's subconscious. *Tsubo* are a manifestation of the *kyo* pattern and may be as deep as the deepest psychological level, tracing far back into one's past. Depending on the skill of the healer, it is possible to reach even the deepest *tsubo* and be able to cure it. This means that shiatsu heals the patient by reaching the deepest levels of the mind, and speedy recovery results after relief of past disorders.

In most cases the *kyo* meridians are deeply buried. However, when empathetic shiatsu therapy is performed on them and the *kyo* is supplemented, the meridians that are empty and deeply drawn inward begin to rise to the surface. The healer must always maintain passive feelings toward the patient when supplementing the *kyo*. However strong the application of pressure needs to be, if the healer approaches the patient with passive empathy, the *kyo* induration reacts by dissolving, and the patient's *ki* is released. A *kyo* induration is the source of every illness. I believe this to be a hardening of negative energy, like karma, which accumulates in the patient's *alaya* consciousness.

In Oriental medicine the source of illness generally seems to be the *kyo* pattern in the meridians caused by a stagnation in *ki*. Harboring negative thoughts and emotions causes *ki* to stagnate. When this continues, *ki* accumulates in the patient's body and mind and forms a lump (the *kyo* induration). The *kyo* pattern is not an indication that the meridians themselves have something wrong with them but that they have become burdened with negative energy (known as *ja-ki* in Japanese) generated by stagnated *ki*. Therefore, the meridians diagnosed as *kyo* are not in themselves *kyo* but indicate a *kyo* induration manifesting symptoms in the various organs positioned on these meridians. In other words, if a *kyo* induration exists, the meridians that carry this burden are diagnosed as the *kyo* meridians. Meridianal therapy following *sho* diagnosis expels the negative energy accumulated in the patient's body and mind, resolves the *kyo-jitsu* pattern, liberates the stagnant *ki*, and restores the patient's health.

Sensing the Patient's Whole Body
and Becoming Passive

Sensing the patient's whole body cannot be achieved through physical application of pressure. It is, more appropriately, attained through an image of support and protection of the patient. Because shiatsu is the application of pressure on the patient's body by the healer's fingers, as far as the patient is concerned, physically the healer's movements are *active*. However, from the point of view of *ki*, it is rather the opposite because the healer's actions are always *passive* toward the patient. Because shiatsu is the act of understanding the patient empathetically, the healer must always approach the patient with unlimited selflessness and a clarity of mind in order to sense the patient's responses. Then, through empathy, the patient's vital force is heightened and he or she acquires the freedom of health and well-being.

Mechanical tools such as the shiatsu roller usually became obsolete soon after their release. Even if these seemed to be beneficial at first, their ineffectiveness was quickly revealed because tools do not have the power of empathy. Likewise, even physical pressure, though temporarily beneficial, has no empathy with life and is not useful for the long-term promotion of health because it eventually results in a hardening of the muscles. The shiatsu therapist has empathy with the spirit of each individual patient's life and can sense that all the energy of the universe and nature dwells within each patient's life. Grasping the sensations of the patient's whole body is related to acknowledging the universal life that dwells therein. *Sho* diagnosis is possible only when this point of view is broadened. This is because actually sensing the meridians and being able to see them clearly means being able to sense the universal life within the patient.

Meridians do not have a physical existence that can be measured quantitatively but are the currents of the phenomenon of life. The flesh of the body can be compared to the actual form or water of a river, while the meridians can be seen as the current. When we look at people with the naked eye, we only see the physical body, just as we only see the water and form of the river. To see the meridians we must look deeper, as though to see the current and not the physical form of the river. The current, unlike the physical body, cannot be understood as something extending between two points. Therefore, sensing the current of the river is not simply perceiving the boundaries visible to the naked eye. It means sensing the currents in the whole natural world: the water streaming down the mountain becomes a river, which flows into the ocean, where the water evaporates and becomes rain, once again falling on the mountain. Similarly, when looking at meridians the healer must realize that the life that dwells within the individual's body is related to life of nature and the universe and that all life is mutually interrelated and in a constant state of exchange: an eternal current without stagnation.

The Significance of Meridianal Therapy

The *kyo* induration in the meridians is an injury to the body of *ki*, and the *kyo-jitsu* pattern continues to form like year rings on trees. The *kyo-jitsu* pattern itself deeply affects a person's posture, movement, and psychological tendencies. As such, it inevitably has a close relationship with the source of each person's life. In the example noted earlier, Large Intestine *kyo* and Spleen *jitsu* are typical sources of the common complaints of stiff shoulders. This *kyo-jitsu* pattern does not simply cause the physical inability to raise the arms: Large Intestine *kyo* can be responsible for psychological states such as a lack of self-expression, and Spleen *jitsu* may be the cause of extreme pensiveness. In other words, the effects of this *kyo-jitsu* disorder are not simply limitations of physical freedom (caused by the stiff shoulder or arm) but also restrictions in psychological freedom. This is to say that people who suffer from such fixation of a *kyo-jitsu* disorder endure a way of life far removed, both physically and psychologically, from their natural state.

Nature provides limitless order and harmony. When people live without generating *kyo-jitsu* disorders through negative emotions and persistence born from their own ego, they live a life of order and harmony with unlimited psychological freedom. Shinran, one of the founders of Japanese Pure Land Buddhism, preached his belief in following the Laws of Nature, which he expressed as a psychological state without judgment in which everything is entrusted to Amida Buddha, who exists at the source of the universe and nature. He preached that all one's actions would naturally be Buddhist deeds from which a perfectly orderly and harmonious way of life is born. In Chinese philosophy this is expressed as "follow but do not exceed your desires," and in Christianity as "the self does not exist without Christ living within." Like Pure Land Buddhism, both Chinese philosophy and the Christian doctrine exclude the element of self-judgment from their separate paths to a greater life.

The difference between the patient's response to the empathetic approach and to the self-centered forceful approach is not unique to shiatsu practice. Those who through the force of their ego have narrow-minded, restricted, and reserved attitudes can only open their minds and express empathy to people who are interested in what they are saying. An empathetic attitude is one that discards the self and tries to become one with the other. In other words, empathy is love, and in love there is no feeling of control of others or one-sided emphasis on the self. What responds to empathy is life; love activates life and life exists through the promise of freedom. Correcting a disorder and relieving the *kyo* induration that injures the patient's body of *ki* is the union of the individual with nature. The patient is released from the bondage of ego and has the potential for freedom and heightened vitality. Tao shiatsu does not only cure illness. Acting as a catalyst in the patient's suppressed subconscious, it helps provide the gift of freedom from a lifestyle that has been restricted by the fixation of a disorder.

The Menken Response

As shiatsu therapy continues, often even after only one treatment, the favorable Menken Response is manifested. This occurs when therapy results in heightening the patient's vital force and expelling the toxins within the body. It allows emotions and ailments that had until then been suppressed to surface and manifest symptoms such as fatigue, drowsiness, diarrhea, or fever, sometimes increasing the pain and often causing abdominal pain. The symptoms that appear as a result of the Menken Response may be similar to those of past ailments. (For instance, patients who suffered diphtheria as children manifest symptoms exactly the same as those of diphtheria.)

The Menken Response may last from a few hours or days up to several weeks, depending on the depth of *kyo*. In severe cases, symptoms such as drowsiness may cause some patients to sleep continuously for as long as one week (waking up only at mealtimes). In cases of fever and diarrhea or when symptoms of a past illness are manifested, patients fall under the misconception that they have become ill. When such symptoms appear after therapy has begun, the healer must first of all determine whether they are due to the Menken Response or are, in fact, due to a true state of illness or wrong therapy. As the symptoms caused by the Menken Response are relieved, the mind and body feel refreshed and healthy. However, when the symptoms are due to wrong therapy or treatment, even if there is relief, the patient never experiences any feeling of rejuvenation or well-being. Often, inappropriate treatment results in damage to the *kyo* in the back, lower back, and neck. Also, treating the *kyo* pattern with one-pointed, consciously concentrated pressure is uncomfortable for the patient, and if it continues, unfamiliar symptoms may appear. This is not a favorable response and will cause deterioration in the patient's condition. Therefore, to avoid detrimental results when treating *kyo*, one must constantly ensure that the pressure is not uncomfortable. If the symptoms that are manifested after treatment has begun do not match those of the typical Menken Response, it is important to consider the possible development of illness.

Before commencing treatment, one must explain the Menken Response to patients and continue to observe their behavior and inform them of their symptoms as they appear. It is difficult to predict the onset of the Menken Response because it can occur rather suddenly at any time between the first treatment and several months into therapy. The Menken Response is not limited to one occurrence only. Just as waves on the ocean are of different strength, the Menken Response continues to manifest various forms and subside again depending on the seriousness of the illness. I have treated one patient for whiplash on three different occasions, taking two years before he healed completely. During this time varying degrees of diarrhea, fever, fatigue, and severe drowsiness were manifested. At times the response was so strong that the patient slept for almost a week. Responses such as drowsiness are the surfacing of fatigue that had until then been suppressed because of too much stress in the sympathetic nerves. Because therapy is heightening the patient's vital force and healing the disorder, the toxins within the body are expelled and the symptoms of drowsiness appear.

Since the patient retraces past experiences in therapy, the Menken Response may manifest symptoms that are similar to previously experienced ailments or emotional states. I believe that this is because meridians are related to the *alaya* consciousness, which lies deep within the normal subconscious. In Buddhism, the subconscious is understood in terms of different levels and the *alaya* consciousness is explained as the eighth consciousness, beyond what is generally thought to be the subconscious (called *mana* in Buddhism). The *alaya* consciousness, also called the "collective conscious-ness," is an accumulation of all past experiences (chapter 1).

Acquiring clinical experience in Tao shiatsu allows the healer to under-stand that *kyo-jitsu* disorders in the meridians form layers or levels like the constant generation of year rings on trees. The deeper the level that carries the disorder, the longer it has been accumulating. As superficial *kyo-jitsu* dis-orders are cured, previously experienced disorders continue to manifest at deeper levels. Generally, in order to cure one level of disorder, it is necessary to perform treatment many times over and the Menken Response often man-ifests when each level is cured.

Manifestations of the Menken Response

1. Expelling Toxins. Symptoms such as fatigue, drowsiness, diarrhea, and fe-ver occur as toxins are expelled. At this stage, the patient should avoid heavy work and exercise, resting as much as possible. Care must be taken because if the patient tries to work, drinks coffee to stay awake, or takes prescription drugs for the diarrhea and fever (mistaking the symptoms for real illness), the release of toxins, which takes place while the body is at rest, is suppressed.

2. Chronic Symptoms Changing to Acute Symptoms. If toxins have been internalized, acute symptoms may become chronic. In such cases, what ini-tially caused the severe superficial pain begins to cause a dull, internal pain. Such pain begins in the arms or legs, moves to the chest or back, and ends up as sharp pain in the abdomen as it moves toward the centermost parts of the body. As the disorder is corrected through treatment, the Menken Response takes over and this process is reversed. In other words, when the pain in the back and abdomen has been relieved it moves to the legs, and as toxins con-tinue to be expelled, the pain continues to move away from the central parts of the body. Conversely, if pain in the legs has been relieved but moves to the abdomen (toward the center of the body), it must be considered to be due to wrong treatment and not the Menken Response.

Another example is the relief of *kyo* pain in the left leg that then moves to the right leg as the condition reverts to its initial state (the *jitsu* pain in the right leg). When chronic symptoms are treated, they always return to their initial state. Stiff shoulders often show a *jitsu* stiffness, and therapy is not complete until the *kyo* that has caused the *jitsu* stiffness has been treated. Treatment stimulates the surfacing of deeply rooted disorders, and healing progresses once chronic symptoms return to an acute state.

The Menken Response may often be very uncomfortable. However, even though at times the patient feels that it is difficult to endure the pain, it never exceeds the limits of the patient's vital force. It is important to consider the patient's psychological reaction to the symptoms of the Menken Response because if patients do not have sufficient confidence and trust in their healer, they cannot endure the symptoms and turn to prescription drugs for the supposed illness. Healers must gain their patients' confidence while making every effort to become people of trustworthy character.

3. Manifesting Past Illnesses and Suppressed Emotions.   Fundamentally, the manifestation of past illnesses and emotions is similar to the surfacing of deeply rooted disorders. Previously contracted illnesses (and disorders) often leave their mark on the body of *ki*, similar to year rings on trees. Through treatment, following the healing of each disorder, the symptoms manifest in the same parts of the body afflicted by the initial illness. Most symptoms that emerge more than once a week after therapy has commenced can be attributed to the Menken Response. One way of determining whether these symptoms are a result of the Menken Response and not true illness is to ask the patients whether they have experienced such symptoms before. For instance, the patient who has frequently suffered from diarrhea or inflammation of the bladder will experience the same symptoms during the Menken Response. It is also interesting to note that as a result of the Menken Response, patients also experience negative emotions suppressed in their past, including their childhood. Therefore, the Menken Response is difficult not only physically but also psychologically.

The Menken Response is a type of cathartic purification and is therefore a very intense period. However, once it passes, the patient feels reborn as though having shed one layer of skin. As disorders are relieved, the patient, while continuing to experience the various phases of the Menken Response, gradually releases blockages of the mind and body. Ultimately, in the ideal Tao shiatsu therapy, the person emerges as a natural being completely free of disorders (in Buddhist terms, "a true person without rank").

The more severe the patient's disorder and the speedier the method of treatment, the more severe the Menken Response becomes. There are some patients who are so surprised at the manifestations that they abandon therapy. Even if the response is not severe, because the human ego has an innate tendency to resist the changes brought about by therapy, the healer sometimes encounters unconscious resistance from the patient. The healer must first of all persist in establishing a relationship of trust with the patient, as this contributes to the release of the patient's vital force. Based on this relationship of trust, the healer is able to provide effective treatment and offer support to the patient throughout the therapy.

Diagnosis in Chinese Medicine

The Relationship between Treatment and Healing

The relationship between treatment and healing is the relationship of mutual faith between the healer and the patient, in which the patient believes in the healer's treatment and the healer believes in the patient's vital force and power of recovery. In Oriental medicine, the human technique of establishing a relationship of faith between the healer and the patient is called the Art of Benevolence (chapter 1). This is not because Oriental medicine relies on a specific placebo effect in therapy, but because it takes medical healing to be impossible without the human relationship between the healer and the patient. This is because the mind affects the body and traditional Oriental medicine has placed great value on psychological healing methods. In other words, healing in Oriental medicine has been called the Art of Benevolence because there has always been strong belief that treatment is inconclusive where there is no relationship of faith between the healer and the patient.

In Western medicine, on the other hand, in extreme cases, surgery is performed after the whole body is anesthetized. This indicates a lack of consideration for the effect of treatment on the state of the patient's mind and consciousness. Differences in prognosis are often indicative of whether patients have been treated by healers in whom they have faith. As can be seen from experiments on the effect of placebos, the only thing gained from impersonal medical treatment is the purely chemical effect of therapy without considering the functions of the mind. Consideration of the patient's psychological state is the fundamental basis for the Art of Benevolence. For instance, if the patient happens to fall asleep during shiatsu therapy it becomes difficult to affect the meridians. Oriental medicine channels *ki* based on the patient's vital responses during therapy, and more emphasis is placed on establishing a relationship of faith with the patient than on anything else.

In *The Yellow Emperor's Classic of Internal Medicine*, the reasons for patients' inability to heal are noted as follows:

1. Selfishness

2. Neglect of body due to financial preoccupations

3. Inappropriate diet and lifestyle

4. Imbalance of yin and yang

5. Inability to take medication due to severe malnutrition

6. Belief in spiritual mediums but not medical practitioners

Therapy develops through a relationship of mutual trust and cooperation between the healer and the patient where there is no medical bias. Healers must improve their skill in order to gain their patients' faith and must cultivate their character in order to have faith in their patients. There are two aspects of gaining the faith of patients and establishing a relationship between healing and treatment. One is the psychotherapeutic technique for the patient, and the other is the healer's personality itself. In other words, the techniques of psychotherapy—acceptance, empathy, and so on—are meaningless unless they are a true expression of the healer's character. In psychotherapy, as in shiatsu therapy, it is inconceivable to exclude the character of the healer, for it is inextricably bound with the clinical psychotherapeutic techniques used. Therefore it is difficult for healers to emphasize psychotherapeutic techniques in their practice without reflecting their own characters. This is because therapeutic techniques are not superficial skills to gain the faith of the patient but are a profound expression of the personality of the therapist.

The Art of Benevolence naturally includes the four methods of diagnosis of Chinese herbal medicine and at the same time incorporates counseling — the modern technique of psychotherapy. The patient's psychological state is excluded in systems of Western medicine because since the discovery of bacteria in the seventeenth century, the source of illness has been looked for externally. However, with the birth of psychosomatic medicine, the need for medicine based on the psychotherapeutic methods of counseling began to be emphasized by some practitioners, and psychiatric units began to be included in hospitals. In the East, however, the four diagnostic methods of Chinese medicine have been part of the medical system for some thousands of years.

The Four Diagnostic Methods of Chinese Medicine

1. Visual Diagnosis. Diagnosis in Chinese medicine begins with visual observation: looking at a patient's whole body and mind and accepting him or her without judging the patient or forming attachments to his or her symptoms. Acceptance of the patient means acceptance of his or her most fundamental behavior revealed through psychotherapeutic counseling. It means magnanimously accepting the disorders in the patient's body and mind without harboring negative feelings or criticism. Some patients do not have faith in their healer and ignore medical advice, which may be irritating. But calmly accepting even this type of patient is one form of discipline through which healers are able to broaden their own therapeutic skills.

Furthermore, whatever their attitude, patients' faith and confidence in their treatment has a positive effect on the psychology of the healer, who must always observe his or her patients' vitality and make their behavior the basis of treatment. The difference between patients who heal easily and those who have difficulty in healing is clear: patients who are appreciative heal easily, and those who lack appreciation take longer.

2. Listening Diagnosis. When the healer has a receptive attitude toward the patient, the act of medical healing takes on the form of listening sincerely to the patient's mind. In the Classics, this is expressed as "the sage who knows by listening." The sage is selfless and has the clarity of the mind to be able to *hear* the patient's actual vital sensations. In other words, hearing² means listening closely without judgment to everything the patient has to express. The quality of listening has traditionally been considered important in the East. In Chinese philosophy, one entire book has been devoted to an explanation of listening. In Buddhism it is said that hearing is the acquisition of faith. In other words, listening closely leads to an understanding of the deeper secrets of life.

The art of listening can also be applied to shiatsu therapy, in which forceful pressure on the patient's body has little therapeutic impact compared to the healer's empathy to the patient's vital response to pressure. Empathy in shiatsu therapy is none other than listening closely with a clear mind to the wavelike moment-by-moment changes in the patient's life. Keiichi Mizushima expresses empathy as follows:

> *Empathy does not mean placing oneself above others and pitying them; it does not mean becoming so involved with the other that you laugh and cry together. Furthermore, it does not mean consenting totally to what is being said or criticizing it. Empathy is the pure state experienced before any such judgment is formed. Empathy is making an effort to feel another's present emotions without value judgment and understanding them to belong to the other and not to oneself.³*

Judging another person through selfish opinions that reflect our own desires and prejudices does not amount to empathetic understanding of that person. Empathy is the unconditional acceptance of another's feelings without affirmation or denial, and it must be based on the recognition that the other's emotions are real. As natural and obvious as this may seem, it is actually difficult to achieve in daily life as well as in the clinic. In general, we can only empathize with others within the bounds of our own spirit (which can be broadened through our own efforts). We have the tendency to judge others through our own standards in order to defend our ego (which is probably why the great teacher Christ also preached, "Judge not, lest ye be judged"). When there are judgmental thoughts in the subconscious, there cannot be

---

2. Hearing and listening are represented by the word *kiku* (to hear) and *kikoeru* (to be audible). This character is made up of the elements for gate and ear and is traditionally expressed as "if one places oneself before a closed gate, what is inside the gate becomes apparent."
3. Keiichi Mizushima, *Kaunseringu Nyumon* [in Japanese] (Tokyo: Dai Nippon Tosho, 1969), p. 117.

empathy and acceptance of others. Judgmental thoughts oppress the other's *ki* and the hinder the purely human-to-human exchange. Empathy in the true sense depends on whether the acceptance of the other is unconditional (in other words, whether there is pure love), and whether egocentric value judgments have been discarded.

3. Dialogue Diagnosis. Visual diagnosis indicates unconditional acceptance of the patient, and listening diagnosis indicates empathetic understanding of the patient's mind 250250(or the wavelike motion of the patient's life). However, acceptance and empathetic understanding are not generated without a positive interest in the patient. A positive interest is the natural expression of inquiry toward the patient. Verbal inquiry is questioning the patient; in terms of Oriental healing, inquiry is therapeutic techniques such as shiatsu.

The shiatsu technique is the complete expression of inquiry toward the patient, and medical healing through shiatsu consists of empathetic understanding of the patient's silent replies (response to pressure). Consequently, shiatsu therapy that does not include such active questioning cannot be called shiatsu in the true sense. Mere finger pressure such as modern massage does not exceed the limits of relaxation and comfort and lacks medical therapeutic value. If healers who learn the Tao shiatsu method do not have the profound understanding that the act of shiatsu is indeed a method of inquiry, they will not be able to practice shiatsu without relying on their own ego, which effectively means they cannot perform meridianal therapy.

Through dialogue diagnosis, a positive attitude toward the patient is not born unless the healer truly desires the welfare of humanity. Naturally, the healer is also human, and human beings are frail, insistent, and envious. One must search intently and recognize the desire for happiness lurking subconsciously behind the envy. If the healer finds faults in the patient's state of health or emphasizes the patient's negative aspects, it is because he or she unconsciously wants the patient to be unhappy. Some ill-natured healers openly emphasize just how much their patient's health is suffering, trying to place the patient under their control by allowing the patient to believe that without their therapeutic skill he or she would not be able to heal. This is fundamentally contradictory to the idea of benevolence and it is one thing healers must never do.

Dialogue diagnosis is born purely from the desire to contribute to the pace of the patient's healthy life. This positive concern for the patient is expressed through an act of therapy such as shiatsu that generates an impartial dialogue between the patient and the healer. In dialogue diagnosis, human respect (or respect for life) is essential, as is the question of how best to improve the quality of human life. It may be said that the worst thing on earth is lack of concern for the suffering of others. People who do not have love for their fellow humans cannot heal them.

It is easy to say that we all must have positive concern for others, but it is very difficult to practice this in everyday life. Most of us, when we read crime and accident reports in the newspaper, are merely relieved that we were not involved. We believe that our own suffering is much more important than the suffering of others. This belief is innate and fundamental to everyone, but under no circumstances must it be allowed to surface in the healer during practice, because patients must always be received with a clear, selfless mind and a positive attitude.

We all have our ego and self-interests. But when we become a patient ourselves, the types of healers we seek are neither those who are concerned only with themselves nor those who cannot face us with a positive attitude. It is impossible for healers to become concerned with patients if they continue to harbor selfish interests in their own daily life, and superficial performances of concern will always become transparent. Healers who wish to face their patients with positive concerns must also cultivate their own actions, words, and deeds and desire the happiness of all in everyday life. In other words, healers must make every effort to become concerned people through words and feelings in their own daily life. Putting effort into each and every thought and idea purifies the subconscious (*alaya* consciousness) and allows the positive concerns to emerge in the way of nature and come to life in the practice of healing.

Redirecting interests from the self to others should not be limited to healers but should be common to all. Even the psychologist Alfred Adler notes that people who are concerned only with themselves are always unhappy, and all suffering is born from among these people (chapter 3). The stronger the feeling of concern toward others, the happier we are, and because such happiness is the basis for the advancement of human life, our future lives are also blessed. As life does not distinguish between the self and others, caring for others means sowing the future seed of our own *alaya* consciousness as care for our own selves.

People who have little concern for others and strong concerns for themselves make firm distinctions between the self and others and are therefore easily afflicted by the negative feelings of fear and anxiety. Fear and anxiety are born from the individualist and separatist mind that does not belong naturally to any part of life. This is why Adler tells his hypochondriac patients, "You will be cured in two weeks, if you continue to think how you can make others happy." Negative thoughts have detrimental effects on the quality of the mind, and because they are manifested as future phenomena, people who, while desiring happiness, have strong concerns for themselves are in fact sowing the seeds of their own unhappiness.

To become happy, we must first of all taste the feeling of happiness. This is the actual sensation of the universal connection between ourselves and nature, born from the joy of knowing that our own life is useful to others. When concern for ourselves is strong, neither joy nor welfare can be gained, because everyone else seems inferior and we cannot generate connection with others or act altruistically toward them. Therefore, in order to be happy and healthy we must begin by desiring the health and happiness of all living things, because behind such desires shine selflessness and infinite purity.

4. Touch Diagnosis. Touch diagnosis means actually touching the patient's body: in other words, empathizing with the patient while positioning the hands ready to apply pressure. In terms of clinical psychology, touch diagnosis may be expressed as observation with concern. This is because no matter how sympathetic and selfless healers are, if they lose themselves totally in their patients they cannot arrive at a diagnosis. Even while feeling the patient's actual life sensations (at the subconscious level) as exactly their own, diagnosis is referred to as *observation with concern* because the patient always remains the *other*. This is where the absolute dichotomy of the union and distinction of the self and other lies. In the Buddhist classics this is expressed as "the vanity of all things" or "the emptiness of all things." This means that the phenomenon of the opposition of all things in existence is the absolute of life; and at the same time, the absolute of life is the opposition of all things in existence. Diagnosis is performed through the healer and the patient becoming one subject but at the same time maintaining the dichotomy of the self and the other.

Visual, listening, dialogue, and touch are the four different methods of diagnosis in Chinese herbal medicine. The essence of these is in fact one and the same concept, explained from four different perspectives. Healers who are truly able to diagnose through visual observation are also able to carry out the other three forms of diagnosis. Heightening one's power of perception in diagnosis means being able to accurately diagnose the *kyo-jitsu* pattern simply by looking at, without actually touching, the patient's body.

The relationship between treatment and healing developed through mutual faith between the healer and the patient is something that goes beyond the healer's nature or psychology. Therefore, rather than being a psychological technique of human relations, these four methods of diagnosis in Chinese medicine allow healers to question their own style of healing. True consideration for the patient is in itself an expression of acceptance of and empathy for the patient, through which the healer fosters the patient's faith and is able to offer relief during the difficult time of the Menken Response and throughout therapy. Therefore, through the practice of Tao shiatsu, healers may cultivate their own character in order to free the universal life deep within their own body and mind.

The healer's attitude toward the patient and the healer's own way of being should be to face the patient with a pure mind without judging the patient's character egotistically, which is equivalent to a respect for life. Harboring good intentions and positive concern for all living things means being desirous of the happiness and well-being of all. From this point of view, whether the therapy is professional or amateur, the promotion and circulation of shiatsu frees people from imprisonment in their own self-centered concerns and restores them to happiness and well-being where there is no distinction between the joys of life of everything and everyone.

If the intended purpose of prayer is people's happiness, then happiness is what is gained. Likewise, if there is empathy with the patient's life from the very first application of pressure, what is gained is an exchange with universal life, which means none other than the purity of thought and the joy of selflessness. The shiatsu method of treatment, which simply uses human hands without drugs or instruments, may be equated to the so-called primitive method of medical treatment, which leads people to the path of happiness and well-being. *Doin* and *ankyo,* systematized with other methods of healing in Chinese medicine thousands of years ago and established as the manual technique offering the utmost respect for life, has been developed to its present form of medical healing technique: the diagnostic system known as Tao shiatsu.

EPILOGUE

e humans cannot help but judge everything through our ego consciousness, and it is consciousness (or, more accurately, reason) that convinces us of the high standard of mental progress we have made. However, consciousness is distinct from all that is innate, and its functions are limited to discrimination and comparison. Through consciousness it is not possible to understand such phenomena as the universality of life, which surpasses comparison and distinction. The fact that the West has reached a state of supremacy in reasoning is not unrelated to the progress of science after its liberation from the oppression of the church. It is thought that historically this supremacy in reasoning was unavoidable. However, it cannot be denied that the pervasive notion in Western thought that the self is distinct from others has generated the advanced materialistic society that is at present destroying the planet.

The burgeoning of logic is a very important consideration in human psychological advancement. As consciousness compares and distinguishes everything, the discriminating mind is said to be as strong as the person's advanced power of reasoning. It is because of this that in extreme cases some people can value life only when they are able to feel superior to others and consequently fall into an inextricable psychological attachment to money, material possessions, and power.

Western logic, with its differentiation between the self and others, is a natural consequence of a Western culture based on distinctions between humanity and nature or humanity and other animals. The destructive direction taken by Western civilization may be the result of holding this logic as superior and denying an even more superior world—spirituality—in the name of science.

Eastern philosophy preaches that the correct path of nature is to be found within the harmony of yin and yang. The union and harmony of the yin spiritual culture of the East and the yang materialist civilization of the West are essential for the future of our planet. However, culture is not the only aspect that must be considered, for the harmony of yin and yang must be searched for in places such as the mind and body and also in religion (yin) and science (yang) and every other aspect of the human race now and in the future.

At present, the planet is in a state of ailment and imbalance. The human race has been excessively selfish, turning scientific technology into weapons. The result of this selfish manipulation of nature is that the planet has fallen into an almost inconceivably unhealthy state. This is the result of emphasis on the acquisition of what is visible and material (*yang*) and the neglect of nature and what is imperceptible and spiritual (*yin*). Living within the union and harmony of yin and yang does not mean the emphasis of one or the other but the pursuit of a holistic nature that balances both. The linguistic origin of the English word *health* is wholeness and holiness. In order for people to be healthy, we need to awaken to a whole and holy nature, and even while maintaining our ego consciousness, we should not live with the illusion that the ego is all there is to the self. We need to discard the view that the material world is the only reality and awaken to a fundamental, universal consciousness.

Even in a world of highly developed scientific technology, the way toward the union of yin and yang for the human race requires the development of a deeply spiritual society and the search for profound harmony between people and the planet. I believe that this may be possible through the harmonious union of yin and yang cultures, that is, Eastern and Western cultures; and that by basing Western materialist civilization on a foundation of Eastern spiritual culture, the road on which they can unite will open.

Pollution and destruction of nature and the environment present serious problems on a global scale for the well-being and survival of the human race into the twenty-first century. The evidence indicates that the violation of any one part of nature disrupts ecological cycles, resulting in the possible destruction of the entire planet. The extinction of species of animals through indiscriminate fishing and hunting is believed to have risen to the extent that it will have a profound effect on world ecology. It has now become essential to urge a change of direction from the present ideology of control over nature (influenced by the progress and application of scientific technology) toward an ideology that sanctifies and harmonizes with nature. This change does not mean that we must deny or discard the scientific technology and materialistic civilization that has emerged until now. But if violation of nature is allowed to continue at the present rate, it will certainly mean global destruction, caused by the materialistic civilization that the human race has itself created.

The essential change of direction must be toward creating a new culture that harmonizes with nature based on a spiritual perspective. The redirection must be toward a culture able to find a more even balance between the spiritual and the material. Without a culture that recognizes that the earth's well-being is the well-being of one form of life, we will continue selfish depletion of natural resources, and as a result, each one of us will have to pay with our health and life for the destruction of nature and the environment. Those involved in scientific technology and development must become aware of the inadvertent destruction that has been wreaked on the planet. For the re-direction of thought and action to take place, it is essential that Eastern ideology form the foundation of science as a new philosophy. It is possible to say that the ever-increasing progress of the materialistic world requires the support of a spiritual culture. This may signify a potentially complementary relationship between Western materialism and Eastern spiritualism.

The facts that many Eastern countries are aiming toward Western industrialization on the one hand and the people of many Western countries are searching for Eastern spirituality on the other indicate that the encounter between the East and the West has already begun. In the Far East, the economic success of Japan through industrialization and, in the far west (the west coast of the United States of America), the development of the new age movement, which is deeply founded on Eastern spirituality, are first steps toward the fusion of Eastern and Western cultures.

The mission for the human race in the twenty-first century must neither follow materialism and selfish exploitation of nature nor overestimate spirituality, as is all too often the case in the East. (In India in particular, through overestimation of the spiritual, material existence is perceived as an illusion—*maya*.) We need to question our tendency for extravagance, be it spiritual or material, as we seek to eradicate poverty and famine from the world and restore the harmony of the planet.

It is essential for medical science, which deals with people's lives, to reconsider the ideology that the physical application of scientific method is the ultimate means of treatment. The human body must be viewed as one part of nature and maintained through equally natural food products and healing methods. Health and well-being should be attained not through drugs and instruments but through insight gained by our own efforts and personal experiences. This does not mean that we should overestimate any particular therapeutic method, be it Oriental or Western. Oriental and Western medicine are both indispensable and complementary to the preservation of every person's health and life, similar to the two wheels of a rickshaw. Western medicine excels in the treatment of all types of contagious diseases and in emergency therapy, whereas Oriental medicine is much more appropriate for treating chronic diseases such as asthma and neurological complaints. The Eastern methods of medical practice and health care, which effectively improve health and strengthen the vital force, must not only exist among a select few but become an asset common to all humanity.

GLOSSARY

ankyo 按橋　Healing through massage and manipulation.

doin 道引　Self-healing through breathing, meditation, *ki* training, *qigong*, etc.

hara 腹　Abdominal area.

ho 補　The character is also pronounced *oginau* in Japanese, meaning to support, supplement, make up (losses), compensate. The *ho* method of therapy, often referred to as *tonification*, complements the *sha* method (see below).

ki 気　Spirit, mind, soul, heart, mood, feeling, temper, nature, energy.

kyo 虚　The character means emptiness, unguarded position, unreal. Also pronounced *munashiku*, make empty, and *uro*, cavity, hollow. In illness and diagnosis, it is a pattern of deficient *ki* energy in the body or the meridians.

jitsu 実　The character means reality, substance, essence, and seed. In illness and diagnosis, it is a pattern of excess of *ki* energy in the body or meridians.

qigong 気功　A self-healing method that uses body movement, breathing, and meditation techniques. Pronounced *kiko* in Japanese and *chigon* in Chinese.

sendo 仙道　"Taoist discipline." The character *sen* (仙) is made up of 人 (person) and 山 (mountain). *Do* (道) means *Tao*. Modern usage is path, way, moral doctrine, technique, art.

sha 写 Also read as *utsuru,* to be projected. In the *sha* method of therapy, *ki* energy is projected away from the parts of the body where it has accumulated in excess. Often referred to as dispersal or calming, the *sha* method complements the *ho* method.

sho 証 The character means evidence, proof, certificate, to prove, to guarantee. *Sho* diagnosis is fundamental to all branches of Oriental medicine. It determines excess, *jissho* (実証), or deficiency, *kyosho* (虚証), of *ki* energy in parts of the body and the meridians.

seiza 正座 The characters mean correct sitting. A traditional Japanese way of sitting on the floor or on cushions by kneeling.

sub-meridians Symmetrical in the body to the main meridians but not mentioned in traditional and Zen shiatsu charts.

tanden 丹田 A point in the center of the abdomen four fingers below the navel, which is the center of *ki* energy in the body.

teate 手当 Means "medical treatment" and "economic support" in modern Japanese. Literally means "the application of the hands." Here it refers to the type of therapy where the healer carries out diagnosis and treatment by using the touch of the hands on the patient's body.

tsubo 壷 The character means jar, pot, hinge, knuckle, one's aim. This is a point of therapy on the meridians.

Index

Numbers in italics refer to illustrations.

abdominal pain, 242, 244
acupuncture, 42, *43*, 49, 87, 144–145, 146, 168, 173, 233
acute symptoms. *See* symptoms, acute/chronic
adaptation, 188
additives, chemical, 22, 152, 182
Adler, Alfred, 152, 251–252
adrenaline, 186
aging, 186–187
agriculture, 8–9, 17, 22
aikido, 35. *See also* martial arts
air conditioning, 189
alaya consciousness, 15, 239, 243–244, 251
alcohol, 164, 190
alimentary canal, 182
allergies, 189
amoeba, 149, *150*
anesthesia, 42, *43*, 165, 246
anger, 44, 50, 74, 152
ankles, 183
ankyo. See *doin-ankyo*
anxiety, 28, 43, 44, 252
appetite, loss of, 182
arms, disorders in, 166, 244
Art of Benevolence, 45, 56, 57, 246, 247, 248
Art of Immortality, 52–53
asthma, 189, 258
astrology, 87
automobile accidents, 184, 188

back ailments, 180, 185, 235–236, 244
back region, and meridians, 176, 190, 232, 243
Basedow's disease, 188
basic whole-body shiatsu, 66, 90, *92–120*, 225, 229, 237
beginners: common mistakes of, 66, 76, 77–78, 84, 170; jitsu technique for, 166
behavior, 149, 171
Benevolence, Art of, 45, 56, 57, 246, 247, 248

Bladder Meridian, 150–151, 185, 187, *206–207*
blood, 183–184
blood pressure, 6, 188
blood vessels, 183–184, 187
bodily fluids, 187
bones, 186
Book of Changes (I Ching), 10, 11, 36, 146
boshin (five color method of classification), 24, 183
brain, 46–47, *47*, 183, 258. *See also* midbrain
bread, 22
breasts, 182
breathing, 58, 179–180, 227
bruises, 184, 231
Buddha Nature, 4, 149
Buddhism: beliefs of, 4, 20, 37, 75, 172, 238, 241, 249; and *sho* diagnosis, 142, 143, 154–155; and subconscious, 15, 243–244; Tantric, 35. *See also* Zen

caffeine, 181, 186, 244
cancer therapy, 42, 44, 58
car accidents, 184, 188
cerebral palsy, 180
chemical additives, 22, 152, 182
chest pain, 244
chewing, 183
childhood ailments, 242
children, 54–55, 72, 149, 171; shiatsu for, 65, *121–139*
chills, 187
Chinese herbal medicine, 6, 7, 168, 169
Chinese medicine, four methods of, 248–253
chiropractic, 51
Christ, 59, 171, 249
Christianity, 4, 42, 58, 241
chronic illness, 68, 153, 234, 244–245
circulation, 184, 187
Classics of Oriental Medicine,

168-169, 173–178; quotations from, 50, 76, 248; mentioned, 24, 49, 54, 68, 181, 186, 189-190
climate, 3, 5, 8, 49–50
coffee, 181, 186, 244
coldness, in extremities, 184, 187, 188
colds, 181, 189
compassion, 48
Conception Vessel, *34, 83,* 89, 190, *216–217,* 227
conformity, 188
consciousness, 13–15, 256, 257
constipation, 181
continuous steady pressure, 68, 70, 79–80, 230
contusion, 161
counseling, 238–239, 248
criminal behavior, 171

damage, to *tsubo* and meridians, 228, 238, 243
defense, 188
depression, 152
Descartes, René, 18
dharma, 53
diabetes, 5, 183
diagnosis, 11, 24; points of, *220;* techniques of, 248–252. See also *hara* diagnosis; pulse diagnosis; *sho*, diagnosis
diagrams. *See* meridianal diagrams
dialogue diagnosis, 250
diarrhea, 143, 181, 242, 243, 244
diet, 22, 23, 152, 181, 247; and meridians, 181, 182, 186, 189–190
digestion, 143, 183, 189
dizziness, 190
Dogen, 35
doin-ankyo, 5–6, 40, 49, 50, 51–52, 259
drowsiness, 242, 243, 244
drugs, prescription, 52, 244

earnestness, 238
echo response, 223, 228
ecology, 257. *See also* environment
ectoderm, 150
elbow pressure, *64*
emergency care, 5, 258
emotions, negative, 44, 152, 239, 241, 245, 252
empathy: and ego, 28, 172, 242; and meridians, 27, 155, 156–157, 171, 237, 238; in all shiatsu, 240, 249, 253
endorphin, 37, 42–43
energy, 2, 19, 21, 37, 39–40, 85, 155, 179. See also *ki*
energy cycle of nature, 5, 7, 9, 20, 148, 155
endoderm, 150–151
environment, 22, 23, 256, 257–258
exercise, 67–68
experiments, 41, 81–83, *82,* 175
eyes, 181, 186

faith between healer and patient, 45, 72, 76–77, 245, 246–248, 253
fatigue, 43, 189, 190, 242, 243, 244
fear, 252
fever, 143, 242, 243, 244
Five Color Method of Classification *(boshin),* 24, 183
fixation, 74, 151, 152, 179, 241
flour, 152
food. *See* diet
form, 155, 240–241
four finger pressure, *64*

gai-tan, 33. See also *sendo*
Gall Bladder Meridian, 118, 151, 189–190, *214–215;* disorders of, 143, 182, 183, 184
gastric imbalance, 182, 189
Gestalt psychology, 13, 17
Governor Vessel, *34,* 89, 190, *218–219,* 227
grasping pressure, *63*
Guthart, George, 84, 163

hair, 186
hallucinations, 185

happiness, 48–49, 79, 251–252
hara, 145, 259
hara diagnosis, 64, 145, *220,* 235–237. *See also* meridianal therapy
headache, 189
healer, 166, 251; attitude of, 76, 143, 239, 240, 250–252, 253; body position of, 80–82, 84, 89. *See also* faith; union of subject and object
health, linguistic origin of, 74, 257
Health and Healing (Weil), 26
health care spending, 22
Heart Constrictor Meridian, 187–188, *208–209*
Heart Meridian, 150–151, 183–185, 188, *202–203*
heel of the hand pressure, *63*
hemorrhoids, 190
hernia, intervertebral, 185
ho. See *ho-sha*
homeopathy, 6
horizontal meridians, 177, 224, *225*
ho-sha, 65, 68–70, *69,* 90, 147, 233, *234,* 259, 260
hospitals, 22, 46
hyakue point, 33, 118, 138

I Ching, 10, 11, 36, 146
Iijima, Kanjitsu, 57
illness: and *kyo-jitsu* pattern (*see also* meridians), 151, 154, 245; in Oriental medicine, 2, 5–6, 19, 46, 52, 238. *See also specific ailments*
image. *See* self-image; visualization
imagination, 185
Immortality, Art of, 52–53. *See also* longevity
immunity, 28, 73
index finger pressure, *64,* 228
individuality, 4, 58–59, 172, 186
induration, 179, 225, 235–237, 239
industrialization, 22, 258
inquiry, spirit of, 250
insomnia, 187

jissho, 67–68, 260. See also *jitsu;*

kyo-jitsu pattern; *sho*
jitsu: definition of, 24, 148, 259; diagnosis of, 144, 165–166, *233;* treatment of, 153, 161, 232–233. See also *kyo-jitsu* pattern
joints, 182, 183
judgment: of self, 241; of others, 249–50
judo, 74. *See also* martial arts
Jung, Carl, 14–15, 172

karma, 15, 46, 239
Katsuta, Masayasu, 163–165
ki, 24, 76; center of, 58, 186–187; channeling, 88, 89; cushion of, *226, 227,* 236–237; definition of, 10, 32, 259; disorders in, 162, 179, 241; and emotions, 50; evidence for, 35, 36, 40–43; method, 84–90; in Oriental culture, 33, 35–36, 58; restoration of, 50, 223, *224,* 235; and *sha* therapy, 233; in *sho* diagnosis, 143, 158; spreading of, 162; stagnation of, 50, 67, 239; universal, 36, 48, 52, 58–59; and the West, 20, 37, 38; yang energy of, 33–34
ki shiatsu method, 84–90
Kidney Meridian, 39, 111, 150–151, 185–187, *204–205*
kinetology, 83–84, 163
Kirlian photographs, 57
Ki Society, 40–41
knee pressure, *64*
knees, 183
kyo, 179, 184, 224; damage to, 243; deep, 229, 230, 234; definition of, 24, 148, 259; depth of, 239, 242; diagnosis of, 144, 154, 157, 158; locating, 155–156, 232; treatment of, 153, 159, 222, 233, 234–235, 241
kyo-jitsu pattern, 67–70, 145, 148–149, 177–178, 244; diagnosis of, 75, 76, 143, 144, 166, 235; in life, 179, 241; and symptoms, 230–231, *231,* 232, 234, 244–245
kyosho, 67–68, 86–87, 260. See also *kyo; kyo-jitsu* pattern; *sho*

Lao-Tzu, 10, 40, 55, 75; and "non-action in nature," 53, 66
Large Intestine Meridian, 111, 118, 151, *194–195;* disorders of, 21, 181, 241
leg pain, 244
lifestyle. *See* modern lifestyle
listening diagnosis, 51, 248
Liver Meridian, 151, 183, 189–190, *212–213*
longevity, 40, 52, 186
Lourdes Springs, 41
love, 49, 242
Lung Meridian, 151, 158, 160, 179–181, *192–193;* disorders of, 181, 184, 185
lymbic system, *28,* 29, 47, 77

macrobiotics, 85
magic, 46, 55–56
mana consciousness, 15, 244
martial arts, 5, 29, 34–35, 66
massage, modern, 51, 250
Masunaga, Shizuto: on medical therapies, 19, 51, 54, 143, 170; on meridians, 149, 169, 173–175, 191; on pressure, 70, 79, 85; on specific disorders, 183–184, 185, 188, 232
materialism, 22, 172–173, 256, 257, 258
maya, 18, 258
medicine: Chinese, four methods of, 248–253; emergency, 5, 258; etymology of, *56;* history of, 168, 248; Oriental vs. Western, 2–9, 16–18, 21, 52, 72--73, 142, 258; philosophy of, 48; Western diagnosis in Oriental, 169–170; union of Oriental and Western, 17, 143, 258
meditation, 46–47, *47*
Ménière's syndrome, 188
Menken Response, 151, 242–246, 253
menstrual cycle, 184
mental preparation, 187
mental vagueness, 188
meridianal diagrams, 159, 160, 170, *192–220*
meridianal therapy, 73, 225, 229–237, *230*

meridians: damage to, 223, 226, 227; deciding between, 158, 161, 163; depth of, 160; descriptions of, 20, 21, 27, 169, 239, 240–241; number of, 173–178, 185, 190; in Oriental medicine, 25, 168, 174; pairs of, 147, 166, 177, 181; perception of, 26–27, 171, 172, 237; and *tsubo, 222,* 222–224. *See also* horizontal meridians; Spiral Meridian; sub-meridians; *and other specific meridians*
Mesmer, Franz Anton, 57
mesoderm, 150
midbrain, 24, 28, 47, 186
middle finger tip pressure, *65*
mind-body relationship, 18, 36, 57, 143, 246; examples of, 21, 44–45, 47
mistakes: common, 66, 76, 77–78, 84, 170; serious, 250, 251
Mizushima, Keiichi, 249
modern lifestyle, 21–22, 23, 79, 171, 186, 190
moxibustion, 7, 49, 144, 173, 233
mucous membranes, 182, 188–189
muscles, 182, 190
mythology: Japanese, 168; modern, 46, 171–72

nai-tan, 33. See also *sendo*
Nakayama, Taro, 56
nausea, 189
neck, 190, 232, 243
neurological ailments, 258
neurosis, 153, 188, 238
nervous disorders, 14
new age movement, 258
"non-action in nature," 8, 53–54, 66
nutrition. *See* diet

obesity, 189
Okada, Kazuyoshi, 43
Omura, Yoshiaki, 163
Oomori, Hideo, 85
One Hundred Monkeys (Lyle Watson), 36
O-Ring Test, 162–165, *163*
Osteopathy, 51

pain, 228, 232, 234, 244–245
palm pressure, *62*
palpitations, 188
pancreas, 183
pericardium, 151
perpendicular pressure, 83
persistence, 186
personality, 148–49, 247
philosophy, 5, 48, 241, 256, 258. *See also* Tao
placebo effect, 37, 42, 45, 246, 247
pollution, 22, 180, 257–258
positions: for whole-body shiatsu, 90–91; healer's, 80-82, 84, 89
posture, 180, 188, 241
prana, 58
prayer, 253
pregnancy, 91
pressure: correct use of, 80, *81,* 158, 226, 228, 240; forceful application of, 69, 71, 75–76, 238, 243, 249; techniques of, *62–65,* 68, 70
preventive medicine, 145
primal sense, 79, 170–173, 223, 228
projection technique *(sha).* See *ho-sha*
psychiatric disorders, 45
psychology, 13, 14, 17, 32, 241
psychosomatic medicine, 19. *See also* placebo effect
psychotherapy, 19, 45, 239, 247
pulse diagnosis, 144–145

qigong, 34, 49, 51, 58, 165, 259

reductionism, 21, 23, 45, 52
relaxation, 47, 72
relaxation response, 159, 160
religion, 4, 49, 55, 58, 171–172. *See also* Buddhism; Christianity; Taoism
respiratory system, 181
response to pressure, 159, 160, 223, 227, 228. *See also* Menken Response
rice, 22, 152
Rogers, Carl, 238
Rules of Health, 6

sages, 51, 53, 74, 248
saliva, 182, 183
schizophrenia, 238
second knuckle pressure, *65*
sei energy, 39, 76
seiza, 260
self-defense, 188
self-expression, 181–182
self-healing, 2, 7, 151
self-image, 44, 47–48
selfishness, 238, 247, 256
self-judgment, 241
sendo, 25, 33, 58, 190, 259–260
sex, 39, 186
sha. See *ho-sha*
shamanistic healing, 55–56, 170
shiatsu: basic whole-body, 66,
    92–120, 225, 229; for children,
    65, *121–139;* definition of, 62;
    descriptions of, 48, 58, 70; his-
    tory of, 84; and mind-body re-
    lationship, 239, 246, 250;
    misconceptions of, 62, 70,
    156; tools for, 240
Shiatsu Meridian Chart (Masu-
    naga), 176–177
shin energy, 39
Shinran, 241
sho, 143, 154, 237, 260; diagno-
    sis, 142, 229; and empathy,
    155, 158, 240
shock, 185, 188
shoulder stiffness, 184–185, 190,
    232, 241, 245
singing, 181
Simonton method, 42, 44, 47
skin, 181, 187
slipped disk, 185
Small Intestine Meridian, 118,
    150–151, 183–185, 188, *200–*
    201
society. *See* modern lifestyle
sore throat, 181, 189
speech, 181
speech impediment, 185
spinal disorders, 180. *See also*
    back ailments
Spiral Meridian, 177, 224, *225*
spiritual healing, 55–56
spirituality, 237, 257, 258
Spleen Meridian, 151, 183, *198–*
    199, 241

sprains, 184
Steiner, Rudolf, 88
sterility, 187
stiffness, 161, 184
Stomach Meridian, 151, 160,
    182, *196–197*
strength, physical, 144, 189
stress, 22, 28, 48, 50, 70, 73, 148;
    and meridians, 185, 186, 187
sub-meridians, 177, 191, 229,
    230, 260
sugar, 22, 152, 182, 186, 189–190
support technique *(ho)*. See *ho-*
    sha
success, 238
sustained pressure, *71,* 71–79, 85
sympathy, 77–79. *See also* empa-
    thy
symptoms, 242–243; acute/
    chronic, 153, 234, 244–245;
    kyo vs. *jitsu*, 232, 235

tai-chi (taikyoku), 10, 51, 66
taking up the slack of the skin,
    85, *86,* 88, 225
tanden, 53, 58, *83,* 89, 186, 227,
    260
Tao, 10, 36, 53, 67
Taoism, 4, 39, 186
teate, 54, 59, 235–236, 260
technology, 22, 23, 257
teeth, 186
tests, of visualization, 81–83, 227
Theory of the Five Elements of
    Yin and Yang, 5, 20, 146–147,
    147, 185
third eye, *165*
thumb pressure, *63,* 68
tongue, 185
touch diagnosis, 154, 156, 252;
    and *kyo*, 159, 161, 162, 235–
    236
touch therapy *(teate)*, 54, 57,
    235–236, 260
toxins, 235, *236,* 244. *See also* ad-
    ditives, chemical; coffee; diet;
    sugar
Triple Heater Meridian, 151,
    158, 182, 187, 188-189, *210–*
    211
trust, between healer and pa-
    tient. *See* faith

tsubo, 70, 71, 154, 174; definition
    of, 222–224, 260; locations of,
    160, 223, 228, 229, 235, *236;*
    and meridians, *222,* 222–224;
    therapy for, 65, 225–227, 228,
    238, 239

Ueshiba, Morihei, 35
ulcers, 182-183
union of subject and object, 7–8,
    25, 51, 56, 69, 78, 171
urination, 185, 187
uterus, 187

visual diagnosis, 228, 248
visualization: of ailments, 47–48;
    and application of pressure,
    80, 81–83, *82,* 227; and *ki*, 40–
    43; and *tsubo*, 223, 226
volition, 185

Watson, Lyle, 36
weapons, 23, 37, 256
Weil, Andrew, 36
whiplash, 188, 243
whole-body shiatsu, 66, 90, *92–*
    120, 225, 229, 237
womb, 187
World Health Organization
    (WHO), 48
writing, 181

yang. *See* yin and yang
Yellow Emperor, 40
The Yellow Emperor's Classic of
    Internal Medicine, 40, 51, 146,
    247
yin and yang, 9–18, *12, 13,* 256;
    and *ho-sha*, 69; and *kyo-jitsu*,
    144, 146; periods of time, 85-
    87, 171, 178, 180
yoga, 29, 34, 35, 58, 83

Zen, 35, 43–44, 58, 66, 67, 75, 238
Zen Shiatsu (Masunaga), 232